Lube Jobs

Lube Jobs

A Woman's Guide to Great Maintenance Sex

Don and Debra Macleod

Jeremy P. Tarcher/Penguin
a member of Penguin Group (USA) Inc.
New York

JEREMY P. TARCHER/PENGUIN
Published by the Penguin Group
Penguin Group (USA) Inc., 375 Hudson Street, New York, New York 10014,
USA • Penguin Group (Canada), 90 Eglinton Avenue East, Suite 700,
Toronto, Ontario M4P 2Y3, Canada (a division of Pearson Penguin
Canada Inc.) • Penguin Books Ltd, 80 Strand, London WC2R 0RL, England
• Penguin Ireland, 25 St Stephen's Green, Dublin 2, Ireland (a division of
Penguin Books Ltd) • Penguin Group (Australia), 250 Camberwell Road,
Camberwell, Victoria 3124, Australia (a division of Pearson Australia Group
Pty Ltd) • Penguin Books India Pvt Ltd, 11 Community Centre, Panchsheel
Park, New Delhi–110 017, India • Penguin Group (NZ), 67 Apollo Drive,
Rosedale, North Shore 0745, Auckland, New Zealand (a division of Pearson
New Zealand Ltd) • Penguin Books (South Africa) (Pty) Ltd,
24 Sturdee Avenue, Rosebank, Johannesburg 2196, South Africa

Penguin Books Ltd, Registered Offices:
80 Strand, London WC2R 0RL, England

Most Tarcher/Penguin books are available at special quantity discounts for bulk
purchase for sales promotions, premiums, fund-raising, and educational needs.
Special books or book excerpts also can be created to fit specific needs. For
details, write Penguin Group (USA) Inc. Special Markets, 375 Hudson Street,
New York, NY 10014.

Library of Congress Cataloging-in-Publication Data

Macleod, Don, date.
Lube jobs : a woman's guide to great maintenance sex / Don and Debra
Macleod.
p.   cm.
ISBN 978-1-58542-561-7
1. Sex instruction for women.   2. Sex.   I. Macleod, Debra, date.   II. Title.
HQ46.M186   2007   2007009880
613.9'6—dc22

Printed in the United States of America
1   3   5   7   9   10   8   6   4   2

Book design by Amanda Dewey

Neither the publisher nor the authors are engaged in rendering professional advice or services to the individual reader. The ideas, procedures, and suggestions
contained in this book are not intended as a substitute for consulting with your
physician. All matters regarding your health require medical supervision. Neither
the authors nor the publisher shall be liable or responsible for any loss or damage
allegedly arising from any information or suggestion in this book.

While the authors have made every effort to provide accurate telephone numbers
and Internet addresses at the time of publication, neither the publisher nor the
authors assume any responsibility for errors, or for changes that occur after publication. Further, the publisher does not have any control over and does not assume any responsibility for author or third-party websites or their content.

To Angela

You were right—a shot of oil does stop the squeak.

Contents

· Part Three ·
Accessories

· Part Four ·
Sexual Intercourse

· *Part Five* ·
Maintenance Coupons

Preface

Y ou're writing a book about *what?*"

"Um, well, maintenance sex," we sheepishly repeat to friends over a casual dinner.

We continue to speak, to elaborate on the book's credibility and relevance in modern relationships, but the faces across the table stare at us in mute amusement as the words *maintenance sex* hang in the air. One of our friends swirls the wine in her glass, then interrupts us with a laugh.

"Remember Brad?" she asks everyone. "He was at me six or seven nights a week." She shakes her head. "He was definitely oversexed."

"You should be flattered," counters a male friend. "What's wrong with six or seven times a week? That's normal for some guys. He wasn't oversexed, he was just healthy."

"You only need to exercise three times a week for health," says another woman. "The same should go for sex. Maybe less, even. Quality is more important than quantity."

The men around the table vocalize a loud collective groan of "Not necessarily."

Meanwhile, we struggle to bring the focus back to the book's philosophy. Maintenance sex is an important issue, we say; it's not a joke. But it's no use. The floodgates have opened, and the opinions and punch lines are pouring out. A conversation formerly filled with intelligent discourse on sexuality and the differences between men and women is now riddled with sarcasm, laughter, and a steady stream of horridly too-personal anecdotes regarding the too-lustful libidos of partners both past and present.

We learn, for example, that when oversexed Brad wanted tending, he would spray copious amounts of cheap cologne "down there" in the hope of tempting his girlfriend to go south. Sadly for him, this resulted in more skin rashes than sexual attention. Donovan lowers the standard of conversation more by revealing his secret maintenance regimen: he waits until his withholding wife is asleep, then slips in a porno and uses her body for friction, staring at the screen until he's finished or she wakes. "Whichever comes first," he says with a smirk. His wife looks at him. "Thanks for not making me get up," she drones.

Maintenance sex has a bad reputation, undeserved, in our opinion. And when it isn't being openly ridiculed, it's being otherwise slandered as the bane of a woman's sexual existence. Unfortunately, there is a stereotypical image of maintenance sex that, despite the jokes, is both sexless and joyless.

What do you picture when you think of maintenance sex? An exhausted woman lying dutifully under her man in the missionary position? Perhaps she reaches out her arms to mundanely read a book or nonchalantly answer a ringing telephone while, with great boredom and heavy sighs, she endures his two minutes of grunts and thrusts. Maybe she throws in an around-the-world eye roll for effect as he announces the approach of his moment of glory.

How romantic.

Well, actually, it can be romantic . . . if you let it be. It all depends on your attitude and your relationship with your partner. If both are positive, there's no reason an occasional nuts-and-bolts sex session—even an inequitable one—can't be part of a deeply loving and mutually satisfying sex life. In fact, maintenance sex saved our marriage.

Anyone who says having children doesn't kill the romance either doesn't have kids or *doesn't have kids*. Try thinking sexy thoughts when your ten-month-old is passing gas in his crib like an overstuffed piglet. Try summoning enough energy to climb on top of your partner at two o'clock in the morning after your three-year-old has marched you into the bathroom for his twelfth "I thought I had to go" session of the night. Try getting in the mood when your five-year-old has even the faintest trace of a fever. And that's excluding the much-feared late-night unexpected and interruptus calls of "Mom, Dad, what are you laughing about in there?" followed by a frantic search for your bathrobes as you hear the pitter-patter of little feet coming down the hall at speeds you never dreamed a size-three, frog-slippered foot could travel.

All parents experience this child-induced celibacy to some degree. Increase the number of kids, and the degree creeps upward as well. We have only one child, so you'd assume we're hanging on somewhere just above room temperature, and today that's probably true. But it didn't start out that way.

We were married less than a year when Debra became pregnant. It was a normal pregnancy, healthy and sex-filled, until one afternoon at seven months when everything changed. Debra's blood pressure skyrocketed to stroke levels, and she was confined to a hospital bed with preeclampsia—without warning, preparation, or negotiation. Without even being able to head back to the office to tie up loose ends or explain the circumstances to the boss or angry clients. Suddenly, it was bed rest twenty-four hours a day, seven days a week. As it turned out, we didn't even make it a week.

Only three days later, at three o'clock in the morning, the fetal heart monitor showed the baby was in distress, which, incidentally, is a more genteel way of saying it was dying. Less than an hour later, Debra lay postoperatively in the recovery room while Don stared at his two-pound son, his bony limbs splayed apart and his red, tissue-thin translucent skin pulled tight over his tiny chest. At least he stared at what he could see of him, for with the tubes and cords wrapped around him he looked more like an insect clinging to life in a spiderweb than a child lying in an incubator.

Our son spent two months in the neonatal intensive-care unit. Because we lived in a city two hours away, Debra had to stay in the hospital with our son while Don went back home to work. Don visited on the weekends and often during the week, making the trek back home at one or two o'clock in the morning to be back in the office by six. Debra spent her days and nights at our son's side, cringing every three hours at the Darth Vader–like suction sounds of the breast pump, and dreading the constant *bing-bing*s of the baby's monitor as it announced even the smallest, most benign change in his heart rate or breathing.

We made it through those months and prevailed. More important, so did our beautiful little boy. But as you can imagine, our relationship took a backseat to everything from baby medications to money worries. Sex was a vague memory.

It was the end of a frozen November when we were finally able to bring our son home from the hospital, right in the middle of a particularly nasty winter during which time every cold and flu virus known to mankind seemed to be thriving. For the next few months, we lived in a state of perpetual fear, for we had been warned by our son's neonatologists and pediatricians that contact with the common cold could lead to pneumonia in his delicate lungs.

Both mom and baby were under medical house arrest—for six months, Debra was unable to take our son to any public place. And her prepregnancy plan to put the baby in day care so she could continue to pursue her career as a lawyer? That disappeared faster than a paycheck in the baby aisle. The risk of pneumonia made day care out of the question, and Debra lost her job. Within the space of several weeks, she had gone from being a professional woman with a day-timer to a stay-at-home mom with daytime television.

But back to the sex.

You'd think that after having suffered through two months of forced abstinence we'd be back at it the first night we were in the privacy of our own bed. Not so. Not the second, third, or fourth nights, either. When Don came home after work, Debra didn't greet him at the door with a kiss; she ordered him to the sink and hovered as he scrubbed his hands, elbows to fingertips, while simultaneously assuring her that nobody at the office had sneezed all day. He was no longer her husband but a potential germ vector.

Fear that your five-pound baby is going to get pneumonia is an antiaphrodisiac. We weren't husband and wife that first month home, and we certainly weren't lovers. We were just two people trying to keep a third person whom we hardly knew alive. Almost immediately, we fell into a sexless pattern of hand washing and worry.

It wasn't until a month after the baby was home, some three months since we'd been intimate, that something shifted. Debra recalls watching a daytime television show about unfaithful husbands and how important sex is to a man and a marriage. As if by design, Don brought flowers home and arranged for Grandma to babysit so we could have a heart-to-heart about how we hadn't been intimate in months, how he was feeling forgotten, and how we were losing "us." Debra didn't wait for another sign. Armed with her disinfectant wipes and hand sanitizer, she once again ventured into the populated world outside her front door, in the direction of the nearest lingerie shop.

Debra admits that our first few nights of sexual intimacy after that period of sexlessness were less than satisfying for her (although Don has quite fond memories of them). It wasn't for another week that she began to feel those old tingles resurface and the cravings begin to return. It was as though the maintenance sex was an appetizer that had whetted her sexual hunger, and soon we were enjoying fine dining like never before.

We also found that our physical closeness was a catalyst to reestablishing our emotional closeness as husband and wife. For us, maintenance sex was a way to connect physically and emotionally during a time we felt particularly disconnected. In the midst of our distractions and distance, maintenance sex was a lifeline that revived our intimacy as a couple. Of course, it's possible that we would have found a nonsexual way to reconnect, particularly since we'd always had excellent communication, but that's not how it happened.

Maintenance sex can play an important part in any long-term loving relationship. Perhaps you and your partner have just brought your first child home and you're feeling overwhelmed and overworked. Maybe you're going through a stressful period at work, or maybe things have simply cooled off over time. Or maybe things are as hot and heavy as ever, and you're just practicing a little preventative care. It is remarkable how many of us share the same experiences and emotions, and perhaps you'll get a sense of this solidarity by reading some of the couples' stories in this book.

Regardless of your situation, we hope you'll come to think of maintenance sex as we do: as a legitimate and romantic aspect of a committed relationship. We also hope that you will find enough ideas, information, and advice in this book to help you explore new aspects of your sexuality as a couple and to enjoy each other's sexual company in undiscovered ways. A good sex life is fundamental to a loving partnership, and great maintenance sex is a splendid and sustaining show of love.

Introduction

Even the most mechanically disinclined woman knows that a car requires regular attention if it is to remain reliable. It needs to have its tires rotated, its radiator flushed, its brakes checked, and its oil changed. Ordinarily, a woman recognizes the importance of this full-body, full-engine attention and is happy to set aside the time and effort to take her vehicle to a full-service garage. She loves the smooth ride she gets as a result, and she and her car can continue their love affair, dodging bumps in the road and exceeding posted speed limits with blissful impunity. Unlike other motorists, she never has to worry about being stranded on the side of the road, hood up, engine steaming, pride and hope fading.

But what about those occasions when a woman is too busy, too tired, or simply too broke to indulge her beloved vehicle in the full-service treatment? What is a woman to do when the sticker on the corner of her car's windshield warns that the oil needed to be changed a thousand miles before, but she doesn't have the time to pamper all of her car's mechanical parts for a full day at a luxury German car spa? Well, she does what all smart, busy women do. She takes it to the corner drive-thru lube station and spends ten minutes in the driver's seat with her tall latte and a courtesy copy of *The Times* while the techies perform a quickie on the oil filter.

Your man is not so different from a machine. He too needs full servicing on a regular basis: he needs his motor revved and cooled with care, his gears greased, and his timing belt changed. Fortunately for you, he doesn't require this level of care every day. Sometimes all he needs is a top-off of gasoline, a quick wipe with a clean cloth, and a slap on his hood to send him on his way. *Lube Jobs* is for those times, times you want to keep his engine running smoothly with drive-thru speed and efficiency. It's for those times he wants sex, but you want sleep.

Even in the healthiest and happiest of relationships, many women find that their partners crave sex more often than they do. The lube jobs in this book are a great way to provide regular maintenance sex. They keep your man satisfied during those times you'd prefer to pass on the passion while at the same time sustaining your sexual connection as a couple.

When it comes to performing maintenance, attitude is everything. It must never be considered a chore: your partner will catch those vibes and will feel self-conscious, guilty, and eventually resentful. Instead of dismissing maintenance sex as an obligation, embrace it as an opportunity to show your man how deeply you care for him and how important his pleasure is to you. By satisfying his carnal needs and desires even when you're busy or not in the mood, you show him that his sexual contentment is a priority for you.

Lube Jobs supplies a woman with a spicy menu of imaginative maintenance sex options she can have at her fingertips when she's running low on creative energy. Using spontaneity and variety as main ingredients, each lube job offers a fresh way to satisfy a man's sexual appetite without serving him a dish of bland bedroom predictability. Some are no-nonsense, no-frills maintenance quickies with no props or prep time whatsoever, whereas others are more elaborate, requiring more time and effort.

Lube jobs also boast full-spectrum content, including seductive scenarios, naughty sexual techniques for hand and oral stimulation, and tips on the use of sexual aids and toys. Some may use visual sexual imagery, while others offer written erotica. One may rely on a sexual frenzy of different positions, while the next may suggest the serenity of sensual massage and hot-stone therapy. A number may take place in the bedroom, but the closet, car, and office aren't off-limits. Several lube jobs can even be incorporated into your daily routine—from the shower to the supper table—so that you can get the job done without veering off schedule.

Cutout maintenance sex coupons have also been included. Place them in your man's keeping, and let him redeem them at his pleasure. With each new chapter, you can expect a unique, exciting, and practical way to maintain your man.

While it is true that maintenance sex is blatant body servicing and your man is the one having all the work done, there's no reason you can't have fun while on duty.

Lube jobs work best when performed with enthusiasm and a good sense of humor. Rather than lying dutifully in the missionary position and staring at the clock, dive into the moment. Challenge yourself to pleasure your partner in new ways and places. Even if your efforts don't always arouse you sexually, they will likely arouse feelings of tenderness and affection that will strengthen your relationship.

The methodology of maintenance is simple: the job should be performed when you're feeling alert, in a way that's convenient, and it should entail a great deal of diversity. Fatigue, distraction, and routine are three reasons women view maintenance sex as a chore. Too often, a woman climbs into bed at midnight, drained from her day and wanting nothing more than to succumb to sleep, only to find that her partner is reaching for her even as her heavy eyelids close. Or she's finally found the time to tackle a nagging project, and he swaggers into the room like a domestic Don Juan, hoping for some action. It is understandable then, maybe even inevitable, that sex becomes one more thing on her seemingly endless "to do" list.

Happily, the solution is an easy one. By planning a playful sexual encounter in advance—when you have the time and the energy—you can treat your man to a fantastic release and avoid the dreaded "get it over with" mentality that can weaken a couple's love life and build damaging resentment. Why let your man suffer through his days, feeling sluggish and neglected? By setting aside even a few short minutes (longer if you like) for his needs and treating him to one of these ready-made lube jobs, you can send him off, feeling rejuvenated and adored. And you can be sure he'll be even more eager to please when you're the one feeling frisky.

It is important to recognize that *Lube Jobs* is intended for devoted couples in strong relationships who already enjoy a mutually fulfilling love life. It is for the sexually healthy woman who is *at times* uninterested in or unable to have sex when her partner is nevertheless keen. Perhaps she's endured a particularly grueling day with the kids, perhaps it's her time of the month, or perhaps she'd simply rather finish that nagging report she brought home from the office before watching a half hour of mindless television to relax. Or perhaps, as was with us, an appetizer is needed to whet the sexual hunger after a lapse in sexual activity.

All couples experience sexual ups and downs during various times of their life together. Such phases are completely natural, and a lube job may sometimes be enough to jump-start a stalled engine or at least to keep it idling during a difficult stretch. *Lube Jobs* is not the book for couples in relationship distress, nor is it intended for women who have prolonged apathy toward sex, who suffer from sexual dysfunction, or who are experiencing serious problems in their personal lives.

We'd also like to say that we are in no way suggesting that maintenance sex replace the joy and bonding that come from mutually fulfilling or long-session lovemaking; however, lube jobs are a terrific way to keep the embers smoldering when the fire can't burn all night. The occasional short but intense sex session, even a one-sided one, can be a powerful part of a couple's love life. The thrill and anticipation of your next encounter—of when or where it will happen and what you will do—will keep your partner guessing and grateful.

The lube jobs in this book will add an invigorating spark to your sex life, while bringing a stronger, deeper dimension to your relationship. You'll be amazed how much smoother your love life will run after just a few quick twists of the wrench. It doesn't take much to keep that engine purring, and the ride is worth the effort.

Part One

Manual
Stimulation

Lube Job #1

◉

Spot-Free Rinse

Close your eyes for a moment and visualize your typical day.

The alarm sounds. You heave yourself out of bed, shower, drive the kids to school, and battle the rush-hour traffic to get to the office on time. You work, have lunch, work some more, pick the kids up, and drive back home, again racing against a city of road-raging, rush-hour drivers who are all fighting the clock as desperately as you are. You cook supper, clean up, pay some bills online, watch a half hour of television, set the alarm, and hit the pillow, and in less than a minute you're flat out, only to be awakened too soon by the six o'clock alarm.

Notice something missing?

Where's your partner?

Presumably he's running somewhere alongside you in this rat race, but the chances are good that when you visualize a typical day, the time spent with him doesn't take up much of the picture. Perhaps you overlooked him somewhere between clearing the supper dishes and paying the bills. Or maybe he slipped your mind because he's downstairs fixing the washing machine while you're upstairs putting the kids to bed. Why is it that the most precious and beloved part of our lives seems to blend into the background of our day's routine, almost as though it doesn't exist at all?

Well, the answer is as simple as it is sad: The daily grind has a way of annihilating any scraps of spare or meaningful time we might inadvertently stumble across from sunup to sundown. And as it does, it silently chips away at the couple time that every relationship needs to maintain intimacy. Too often, that leaking dishwasher takes precedence over couple time (sometimes even when the relationship is in as poor condition as the appliance!). That's why every now and then, we need to push a towel under the dishwasher and let it leak at will, as we take our partner by the hand and show him he's more important than a small puddle on the kitchen floor.

Fortunately, when it comes to couple time, quality is more important than quantity. That small but mighty realization was something that Angela, a twenty-eight-year-old wife and mother of two small children, says has made all the difference in her marriage: "I used to think we needed a vacation, a physical break from our daily routine, to reconnect and get the spark back," says Angela. "But now I know it's the everyday little moments that count more than the yearly couple's getaway, especially since the yearly getaway tends to skip a few years once you have kids."

"It's important for a couple to incorporate their own special, intimate routine into their larger daily routine," advises Colin, Angela's husband of seven years. "It shouldn't just be about who's going to take the trash out or who's going to mow the lawn. It has to be about the two of you experiencing life together, not just dividing up the labor. If you can get into that mind-set, you've got it made."

Angela and Colin, though happily married, admit that for years they suffered from the curse of modern couplehood—that passion slayer—called the roommate rut. Perhaps it's inevitable that every couple dips into that sexless ditch every now and then. Considering the countless mundane demands we all must deal with every day, it's no wonder that we often find ourselves reaching for a ringing telephone more often than for our partner.

"I'd go days without even looking into Colin's eyes," says Angela. "It's not that I didn't love him—I've always felt very deep love for him—but sometimes I got so caught up in all the things I had to do, that I just looked right past him. He'd be leaning against the counter with his arms out to hug me, and I'd walk right past him to phone my son's coach and find out what time the game was scheduled for next Saturday."

"There was zero spontaneity," Colin adds. "If I wanted sex, I knew the routine, and I knew I wouldn't get it unless everything was done: the kids had to be sleeping, the coffeemaker had to be programmed, lunches had to be in the fridge for the next day, the cat had to be out, the laundry hamper had to be empty, and Angela's clothes had to be laid out for morning, and then she had to brush and floss her teeth and wash her face. If that routine was completed, in order, I stood a remote chance of getting lucky. It didn't happen nearly as much as I wanted it to."

> No time for couple time? Go through your daily duties to see which chores might be more enjoyable with company. Share a longer sit-down breakfast, work out together, walk the dog hand in hand, or wash the supper dishes side by side.

"We really were like roommates for a while," says Angela. "When Colin would come home after work, I'd hand him a bag of garbage instead of greeting him with a kiss. He was just a helping hand, not a husband."

The turning point came one night when the almighty routine was unexpectedly broken. As she stood in the bedroom folding laundry, her teeth still unflossed and her face still unwashed, Angela heard the strangest, most unusual sound: running water. Colin was in the shower, but it was late evening, and his routine was to shower in the morning. It made no sense. Angela went to investigate.

"I slid the shower door open and my jaw dropped," says Angela. "Colin's back was to me and he was leaning against the wall with one hand. The other hand was occupied . . . he was masturbating. It was the first time I'd ever caught him doing it, and I was really shocked."

"I was mortified," admits Colin. "Totally humiliated. Then that feeling gave way to intense anger. I slammed the shower door closed and yelled at her to mind her own fucking business. I don't even know what that meant; I just know I was embarrassed and frustrated, and furious. That was the first and only time I've ever spoken to Angela like that. It was completely out of character for me, but I felt like I was at the end of my rope."

Stunned by her husband's angry outburst, Angela stood outside the shower and stared at the closed door. She felt her own anger flare in response to his words, and she knew the situation could easily spiral into a major battle if she reacted in kind. She struggled to keep her cool as she quickly analyzed the situation. Her husband, whom she knew she had been neglecting for weeks, had been reduced to a covert masturbation session in the shower.

She pictured the unfolded clothes in the laundry hamper. She thought about her imperfect oral hygiene. She visualized Colin sneaking off to gratify himself while she, oblivious and preoccupied, folded socks in the next room. She decided to do something drastic, something big, something so far out of character that she was almost unrecognizable to herself. Without giving herself time to change her mind, Angela quickly took off her clothes and left them in a heap on the floor as she stepped into the shower.

"I literally could not believe my eyes when Angela got in the shower," says Colin. "I remember her exact words. She said, 'Never send a man to do a woman's job.' She pressed up against me and proceeded to give me the best hand job I'd ever had. I went from red-faced anger to pure joy in seconds flat. It was like all my stored-up frustration just went down the drain with the water."

"That was a real eye-opener for me," says Angela. "Seeing Colin like that. I felt like the worst wife in the world, and my heart just broke for him. In that moment I realized how much I'd been neglecting him. I remember just forcing myself to get into the shower, to forget about the things I hadn't done yet, and to do the most important thing of all, which was to be available when my best friend needed me."

Showering together has now become part of Angela and Colin's daily routine. Every morning, they grab their towels and head into their private suite—which they had renovated to include a large walk-in shower stall—and lock the door behind them, leaving the kids to pour their own breakfast cereal. It's their quality couple time, and they have it every single morning, before they have their coffee.

> **When you finally find that precious but elusive couple time, don't waste it talking about work, the kids, or (*egad!*) the bills. Keep the conversation focused on you as a couple, such as how you met, your favorite vacation, and your dreams for the future.**

"Sometimes we fool around, sometimes we're all business. Either way, it's our special time together. And quite often it's the only time we have all day to enjoy each other's bodies and closeness," explains Colin. "It's important. It reminds me that Angela is a sexy woman, and I want her more than I ever did. And it keeps us feeling close, so she's interested in sex more than she ever was. Once you stop being physically close, you don't see the other person as a lover, and you start drifting apart emotionally."

"And that's the beginning of the end," warns Angela.

Angela and Colin, though burdened with the same daily demands as many other couples, realized that they did not need a physical break from their routine to reestablish their loving connection. Ultimately, they found their way out of the roommate rut by working with their routine instead of working against it. Since they both had to shower in the morning, not only did they reduce the early morning stress of fighting for the bathroom, but they also found a way to transform this ho-hum function into a fun, intimate activity that each day served to reaffirm their emotional and physical connection before they headed off in their separate directions.

When it comes to maintenance sex, this couple's shower solution holds particular potential: it's fast, it's fun, and it's effective. And there's no clean-up! The shower can be a very sexy spot to share some quality couple time. The sight of soapy water running over his woman's bare breasts and between her legs can work a man's libido into a rich lather, while the nakedness, warmth, humidity, and calming atmosphere make it a space that's charged with sensuality.

For best effect, lower the lights. You can either light the room with candles or install a dimmer switch for those wet erotic encounters. For better or worse, many women find that they are most at ease with their bodies when the lighting is soft. And since you'll really be working those feminine curves of yours in this lube job, you want to be as confident as possible in your own soapy skin.

In the shower, be sure you have soap, a thick washcloth, a loofah, and some hair conditioner. There are some mint body/shower gels that leave a delightful tingling effect on the skin, and if you can find one of those, so much the better. This lube job is highly sensual and the more textures and sensations you and your partner can play with, the more you'll both enjoy the experience.

> ✳ A shared shower facilitates total body contact, something that many women need in order to feel intimate and become aroused.

When you sense your man's gears are grinding too hard and you know he's in need of a little maintenance, either join him uninvited in the shower or take the initiative and ask him to join you for one. You'll get him aroused just from that! As he stands at attention in the shower and waits for you to hop in, give him a preview by slowly peeling off your clothes in an impromptu striptease. Don't worry about pulling any fancy pole-spinning antics (ouch!), just let him enjoy the sight of his woman's naked body being tantalizingly revealed in front of him. He'll be an easy audience to impress, so snake out of those panties as naughtily as you can and have some fun being a one-woman show.

Step into the shower and, with great exhibition, reach for the soap or shower gel and begin to lather up your body—every inch of it—as your man eagerly watches the sudsy water cascade over your breasts, down your stomach, between your legs. Use your warm, soapy body as sexy bait by gliding your hands over the curves of your breasts, then slipping a hand between your legs to clean your most private area. Most men haven't spent a lot of time watching a woman wash herself "down there," so prepare for yours to be mesmerized by the sight. Play it up for full effect by keeping one hand between your legs while the other continues to glide over your breasts.

Stand under the water to rinse the soap off your body and again reveal your naked skin. If you have a detachable showerhead, you can prolong the rinse cycle by moving the showerhead all over your body, both to wash away the soap and to let your man soak in the sight of the water spray on your skin. Spread your legs (you can even lift one leg onto the side of the tub) and bring the showerhead close to your vagina, letting the spray cascade over your labia while your partner watches. If you're feeling particularly exhibitionist, slip a finger into your vagina.

Ask your partner if he would be kind enough to give you a second wash, back and front; you're just so-o-o dirty! Not only will this prolong your shower session, it'll kick his libido up another notch as he delights in the feel of your soapy skin under his hands. Ask him to wash your breasts and between your legs and tell him how good it feels to have his strong hands touch you in those soft

> **If you're tired of your man's immediate postcoital catnap, try a cool after-sex shower to rejuvenate rather than relax. It'll keep him up for round two.**

places. Rinse yourself off under the water or give your man the detachable showerhead and ask him to do the honors.

Now it's your man's turn to get squeaky clean. Have him turn around and face the shower wall while you stand behind him and lather up his back. Move from his back to his shoulders, then down his arms. Wash his bum and down his legs to his feet, then ask him to spin around so you can wash the front of his legs, moving up to his groin but not yet touching it. Soap up his chest, shoulders, and arms, taking your time to let him fully enjoy the feel of your hands moving so seductively over his wet body. Use the loofah to give him an invigorating body scrub before rinsing him off.

Once his body is spot-free, lather a thick washcloth with soap and get busy scrubbing his man parts. Use the soapy washcloth to clean his upper and inner thighs, then his pubic hair, and finally his testicles. Lift his scrotum with one hand and gently scrub underneath it with the other. Move the cloth very lightly over the shaft and tip of his penis until he is hard. Rinse his genitals off—again, a handheld showerhead would feel exquisite on his penis as the stream of water pounds it ever so tenderly at point-blank range.

Now that your man has experienced the relatively "rough" sensation of the washcloth against his penis, a smoother touch is in order. Take a handful of hair conditioner and slowly, very slowly, stroke his shaft from tip to base and back up again. Squeeze as hard as he likes and gradually pick up the pace until you've reached a good pumping action. When you see he's getting caught up in it, slow down and let up on the pressure around his shaft.

Rinse your partner off. If you have a bottle of mint shower gel, now's the time to use it. Rub it all around his groin area and then rinse it off to let him experience the tingling effect for as long as it lasts. A word of caution: Be careful when you apply any new product to your man's skin and/or genitals. If your man has sensitive skin, stay on the safe side and use his regular soap or a personal lubricant in the shower.

> A silicone-based lube is necessary for watery sex play, since the more popular water-based lubricants will disappear in the water.

The final cycle is now about to begin. Give your man a wet kiss on the mouth and then take another handful of the hair conditioner and use it as a lubricant to finish this lube job. Tighten your hands around his shaft and pump him at a pace and rhythm that will bring him to orgasm, at his pleasure.

This lube job is a great choice for women who want to find a convenient yet sensual way to incorporate quality couple time into their daily routine. It's up to you whether you use shower power for spontaneous, as-needed tune-ups, or whether these sexy sessions become regularly scheduled events to prevent relationship erosion. Maintenance sex has never been so steamy!

Lube Job #2

●

The Jump Start

Naomi and Kurt are a couple who find themselves in the sandwich generation of people caught between caring for children and aging parents. They're both in their midforties, together for over eighteen years, with two teenage kids at home, another away at college, and two sets of parents in declining health. Although their relationship was a happy one, their sex life had in recent months come to something of a standstill: the consuming distraction of Kurt's acutely ill father and the financial stresses of his medical and hospice care had put an understandable damper on romantic thoughts. It's a situation many long-term, middle-aged couples are either currently facing or will eventually face.

Because Naomi worked part time and because the tasks were too emotionally painful for Kurt to carry out, the many details surrounding Kurt's father's care fell to her. It was a busy time for them, and caring for both parents and children left them little time to focus on themselves or their intimate relationship. It used to be that they'd crawl into bed at night and share some sweet pillow talk. Now they talked about the rising cost of their son's tuition, the birth-control pills Naomi found in their teenage daughter's purse, and Kurt's dad's latest laboratory results.

But their growing cares didn't cause Kurt's testosterone levels to decline, and Naomi began to sense that he was feeling sexually neglected, although neither of them seemed to have the energy to do anything about it. Often when they lay in bed together at the end of a long, demanding, emotionally draining day, Kurt would appear affectionate but would fade off to sleep before an equally exhausted Naomi clued in to his sexual cues.

Although she did not feel the same drive during this time as Kurt did (in fact, sex was the last thing on her mind), Naomi came to realize that her husband's sexual needs were not being met. Knowing that Kurt would never pressure her, particularly after all she was already doing for him, Naomi decided that the kindest and most loving thing she could do was to take the initiative and give him what he didn't have the heart or the energy to ask her for.

Naomi decided to take matters into her own hands, so to speak. In addition to the emotional turmoil she and Kurt were experiencing, she knew that their lack of sex was largely due to simple exhaustion. Since the day drained too much of their energy, she knew that she would have to get a jump on it; that is, she needed to jump-start the day if she was going to jump-start Kurt.

The next morning, Naomi woke up early and sprinted into the bathroom for a quick shower before diving back under the sheets, wearing nothing but skin and perfume. She whistled suggestively to wake up Kurt and then asked

> **While stress is unavoidable (some of it is even good), a chronically high level of stress can act like a cold shower when it comes to sex. Don't adopt stress as your lifestyle. Find ways to incorporate stress-busting routines into your relationship: exercise or practice yoga together, share a bath, give each other back rubs, or pick a good book to read and discuss in your own book club for two.**

in her most sultry, sun's-up voice if he'd like to work up his appetite before breakfast. It took a moment for her daybreak temptation to dawn on him, but when it did, a bleary-eyed Kurt sprang to life even before the automatic coffeemaker did.

Naomi's efforts, though minimal, meant the world to Kurt. He realized that his wife still noticed him, still cared for him, and was still willing to take the time to pleasure him despite their hectic schedules and the fact that she wasn't experiencing the same sexual drive that he was. For Kurt, the maintenance quickies were escapist moments of sheer sexual pleasure and a much-needed break from his cares and grief. Because they usually occurred in the morning, before their days exhausted them, they were bright interludes during a dark time.

For Naomi, maintenance sex was not a chore or a duty; it was a gift of love and understanding from a woman to a man. She never approached it as an obligation, and she never acted as though it was too much work. And, just as important, she never performed any sexual act or activity she was not comfortable with. On the mornings that she simply didn't want intercourse, she instead treated Kurt to the best hand job she could perform—and he never complained.

Of course, maintenance sex didn't solve all their problems. It didn't stop Kurt's father from passing, it didn't stop them from worrying about their teenage son driving too fast, and it didn't stop the bills from coming. But it did ensure that during this difficult but temporary period in their lives, their friendship endured and sexual intimacy didn't slip through the cracks. And, as naturally as a river flows to the sea, their lives eventually slowed, their worries lifted, and the early morning quickies gave way once again to the late-night marathons they had always enjoyed.

Naomi's winning logic—to get the job done before the sun comes up—is as practical as it is effective. Exhaustion is the enemy of many couples, and if you're one of them, why not make use of that precious A.M. energy for sexual purposes? As we all know, fatigue is one reason women often regard maintenance sex as a chore. But by taking care of business first thing in the morning, before your day takes over, you'll have the energy to show your man a good time and to make sure he wakes up on the right side of the bed. His motor might be more in need of a jump start than you or he realizes.

As we all know, men often awaken in a state of partial arousal. What could make a quickie easier? Your job is half-done for you, so you might as well take advantage of it and pluck him while he's ripe for the picking.

On the evening prior to this morning quickie, set your alarm for fifteen minutes earlier than usual and stash some

> The easiest way to fight stress is also the most enjoyable. Sex releases powerful endorphins that relax the body, soothe the mind, and improve the quality of our sleep.

personal lubricant nearby. (Water-based lubes are the most popular, since, among other reasons, they feel natural and wash off easily.) The moment the buzzer sounds or the music blares, climb out of bed to prevent the ever-tempting snooze button from seducing you back to slumber. Turn off the alarm and let your man drift off back to sleep while you freshen your breath and body in the bathroom. Strip off your pajamas and stand completely naked in the bedroom doorway, looking as strikingly sultry as possible as the sunlight filters through your bedroom window. You're going for sexual shock value.

Wake your partner with a suggestive "good morning." When he notices your gorgeous form in the doorway, saunter toward him, pull back the sheets, and take matters— that is, his manhood—into your own hands. As he lies amazed on his back, tease and tickle his penis and testicles (over the top of his underwear, if he's wearing them) just briefly before dragging your fingertips up over his stomach and chest and down each of his arms.

Return your attention to your man's groin. Gently pinch the shaft of his penis and cup his testicles in your hand, again over his underwear. Rub his penis and testicles with the palm of your hand: if he isn't wearing any underwear, you can slip the sheet over his genitals to use the friction of the fabric to your advantage. When you wish, you can ask him to snake out of his underwear so he is completely naked.

Lavish your partner's shaft with featherlike strokes from your fingertips. Stroke the entire length, then stop and lightly massage it with tiny circles. Your strokes will have to be very gentle, since you don't yet have any lubrication to be firm. Stop stroking and simply apply pressure to various points along his hardness with the pads of your fingers. Since you don't want him to become accustomed to any one feeling or motion, make sure that your touches and his sensations are unexpected and unpredictable.

Place your palm on the *glans* (head) of your partner's penis and press down gently. Now turn your hand, as if unscrewing the lid off a jar. Do this only a few times before turning your attention elsewhere. To change what he's experiencing, lightly tug at the soft pubic hair at the base of his shaft. You want his entire groin area to feel alive.

Now take his testicles in your hand and bounce them in your palm. Tickle and scratch the *perineum* (the area under his scrotum, between the sac and his anus). Apply gentle pressure as you pull his scrotum away from his body and then roll it up the underside of his shaft. Squeeze to apply heartbeat-like pressure pulses of pleasure to his testicles, and, as you do, be sure to tell him how incredibly good his genitals look and feel.

Retrieve the lube from under your pillow or wherever you've stashed it, and warm some between your palms. For an unexpected sensation, you can add a sexy twist to your hand job by using a warming lubricant to heighten your man's experience. These are available at all sex shops and

That's a powerful peppermint! It's believed that peppermint can improve the mood and rejuvenate the body. The next time you feel those late-day slumps coming on, pass on the caffeine and reach instead for a cup of peppermint tea. And to fight exhaustion in the bedroom? Try peppermint aromatherapy instead of floral or fruity scents and a light peppermint body spray in place of your usual perfume.

even some drugstores. They're also the perfect first purchase if you're new to adult novelty stores—they're inexpensive, nonthreatening, and you won't need to ask the salesperson how to use them.

Downstroke your partner's shaft with warm, well-lubricated hands. This initial stroke should be strong, slow, and purposeful. It's the first time this morning that his penis has received this level of direct and sustained attention, and the effect should be a powerful one, particularly when the warming sensation kicks in. Wait a moment to get the full effect, and then pump his penis a few times using both your hands.

Stop stroking. Make an O with the index finger and thumb of one hand and place the O on the head of your partner's penis. Push down so the glans squeezes through the O of your fingers and then slide your fingers down his shaft until your index finger and thumb form a tight ring at the base of his penis. If you wish, you can slide your fingers over and then under his testicles to form the ring under his scrotum instead, although your fingers may not wrap completely around this area. The idea is to steady his genitals and provide a sort of natural penis ring that will increase sensation.

As one of your hands steadies your partner's penis, use your other hand to apply upward-only strokes to the shaft. As his shaft becomes more turgid and sensitive, add variety to your upward strokes by occasionally sliding your thumb or palm over the glans. For additional sensation, with your stroking hand in the shape of a claw, hook your fingertips under the coronal ridge (the ridge around the head of his penis), and pull up.

When you're ready, release the ring around his genitals but maintain the O of your index finger and thumb. Begin to stroke his shaft up and down with the O ring. When you're on the downstroke, use your other hand to twist the head of his penis, again as if you're unscrewing the lid of a jar or turning a dial. It takes a little coordination, but you'll get the swing of it. And practice makes perfect.

Vary your motions and rhythm to keep your man guessing and gasping. For example, you can rub his penis between your palms as if starting a fire. When you downstroke him, be sure to press down on his scrotum as you reach the base of his penis. And don't forget his testicles. Many men love to have them stimulated at the same time the penis is

> **Feeling sluggish? Sit up straight. The more you slouch, the harder your body must work to deliver oxygen to your brain; proper posture can therefore fight fatigue.**

being tended to, so use your free hand to softly squeeze his scrotum and fondle the underside with your fingers.

When you're ready to make your partner's orgasm build, adopt a regular, predictable rhythm to stroke by. Use the pace and amount of pressure that he likes, and pump his penis up and down. You don't need to do anything fancy at this point; slow and steady can make his buildup very intense. As you stroke, slide your hands all the way up and down his shaft from the head to the base.

If your hand coordination and aim are good, let his penis pop out of your grip entirely on the upstroke, then slide it back in for the downstroke. This will mimic the feel of total vaginal withdrawal and penetration. However, if you're not completely confident you have the coordination to slide his penis back into your grip without missing the mark, don't risk it; stop at the head of his penis on the upstroke, then go down again. You don't want an ill-timed "oops" to interrupt the wonderful momentum he's building at this point.

Allow your partner to climax and keep stroking him as he comes. Keep stroking afterward as well, although with less pressure. He may or may not want you to touch the head of his penis, as some men are ultrasensitive here just after they come. Gently squeeze and massage his testicles, then lift them and scratch the area of his perineum to let him bask in the afterglow of his early-morning orgasm. There, the job's done.

However, if even the negligible amount of preparation and effort this scenario entails is too demanding before you've had your three compulsory cups of caffeine, you can try another A.M. approach. Before you go to sleep the night before, stash some lube within your reach but out of sight. The moment the alarm goes off, turn your back to your partner and discreetly warm some lube between your palms. Roll back over to face him and plant an innocent good-morning kiss on his cheek while simultaneously slipping a guilty hand down to his penis. Your partner won't be expecting this rush of pleasure, and it won't take much effort for you to gently caress him to full attention.

Studies show that men have their sexual peak in the early morning hours, while women peak at night. How about a compromise? When you find yourself in the throes of three-A.M. insomnia, try initiating sex with your partner instead of watching late-night television. He'll think he's dreaming, and you'll power down enough to fall asleep.

If you like, you can bring your man to climax under the warmth of the sheets; you won't even have to suffer the chill of the early morning air to get this lazy lube job done. Tell him to look down and watch the blankets move over his groin as your hands are hard at work under the hood. After all, sometimes what we *don't* see is as erotic as what we do see.

Now congratulate yourself on a lube job well done and head for the coffeemaker and the croissants. With only minimal effort, you've managed to jump-start your relationship and your day. And no doubt it'll be a day full of fond memories of your erotic early riser.

Lube Job #3

⬡

Power Polish—For Bad Girls Only

You know that scene in the porno where the guy's about to ejaculate and three hungry women surround him, jostling for point-blank position and smiling greedily, batting their five-pound jet-black eyelashes the whole time, as he plays fireman on their faces? You know, the money shot. The facial. It's quite the performance. And the Academy has the gall to pass over these hardworking ladies for Best Actress? Not even a nod for Best Supporting? For shame.

The money shot is a must in adult films and can take any bodily angle: the facial, the pearl necklace, the breasts, tummy, ass, wherever. And while many female porn viewers don't particularly like it (count Deb in), it's a necessary element for men. Men are visually stimulated, and although most straight men won't line up to watch another man ejaculate, they may enjoy watching a woman take what's coming to her . . . so to speak.

Yet as common as the money shot is on set, it's not as popular offstage, in the bedroom. Although a man may

> The term *money shot*, which was once widely used in mainstream filmmaking to describe the movie's most expensive sequence, is now primarily associated with the pornographic film industry and the act of a man ejaculating on a woman's body. It is used to indicate the end of a scene and to show that the actor really reached orgasm.

want to at least try ejaculating somewhere on his wife or girlfriend's body, some women find the idea demeaning and refuse to entertain it.

"I've checked everywhere," says Isabelle, twenty-eight, "and I haven't found a bull's-eye anywhere on my body. So why would I let my boyfriend use me for shooting practice? I think if a guy wants to jerk off on a woman's body, he sees her as nothing but an object, and he's probably watched way too much pornography. It's a power trip for guys, and it's all about his pleasure. Any woman that lets herself be degraded that way probably has self-esteem issues."

But not all women are so adamant in their opposition.

"It's kind of ridiculous, but it's no big deal," says Katelyn, forty-two. "My hubby will ask me to let him do it every once in a while, and I don't mind. Sometimes it turns me on. You don't usually get to see it since it's usually happening inside, so it's exciting to watch."

And what about being degraded, as Isabelle believes?

"I don't think letting a man come on your body is inherently degrading," Katelyn says. "How is it any less degrading than letting him come inside? It all depends on your relationship. I do think some women let men degrade them, but that's something in them that's lacking, and some women are so hypersensitive about sex that they find anything but the missionary to be immoral. I don't feel degraded when my husband uses my body for sexual pleasure. Women should be more concerned with *whom* they're doing it instead of *what* they're doing. Any sex act with someone who doesn't love you is degrading, but if you're with someone who respects you, anything goes."

"There's something really taboo about doing it," adds Frank, thirty-nine, Katelyn's husband of ten years. "It sounds dirty, but there's something about watching it come out of me and land on her skin that really turns me on. It adds an incredible visual dimension to the sensation of an orgasm that you don't usually have. I especially like it when it lands on her breasts . . . It rolls down the sides, and makes her body look shiny and so erotic. Nasty!"

Without a doubt, the "nastiness" element factors greatly into the money-shot debate. After all, if the bad girls of porn are doing it, should I, a respected wife and mother who doesn't let her bra straps show in public, be doing it, too? Only you can answer that question, but it's one that at least warrants consideration. If your loving partner wants to watch the hidden mysteries of his ejaculation unfold on your tummy, why not watch with him? You might be surprised just how sexy the show can be.

You've heard this kind of thing before: "Men want to go to bed with a virgin and wake up with a whore." "A man wants an angel on his arm but a devil in his bed." Basically, they want it all: during daylight hours, they want a good girl whom Mom would approve of, but when night falls, they want her to morph into a bad girl whose sexual boundaries can't be seen with the naked eye. So why not push some boundaries and explore the various facets of your and your partner's sexuality?

This lube job is ideal for a night you're feeling naughty but not in the mood for oral or vaginal intercourse. Encouraging your man to ejaculate on your body adds a nasty visual and mental twist to the standard hand job, thereby elevating regular maintenance sex to rapturously raunchy heights. Combine the money shot with some dirty talk to really play the bad girl and bring out the bad boy in your man.

> A cream pie is a money shot in which a man ejaculates inside a woman's body—in her vagina or anus—rather than on it. The camera captures the magical moment with a close-up of the semen dripping out of her body.

Climb into bed naked, lube hidden nearby, and summon your partner to the sack. When he joins you, spend some time complimenting him on his impressive sex drive, and tell him you're longing to give him some well-deserved pleasure. You know he's a man who has needs, and you can't wait to fulfill them. Kiss and caress him for a while, moving your hands all over his bare body before focusing on his groin. Comment on how good his cock feels, how big and heavy his balls are, and how masculine his pubic hair feels. As he hardens, respond by touching him more eagerly.

Tell your man how lucky you feel to have such a sexy man in your bed, how so many women would love to be lying beside him, and how his body makes you want to do all kinds of nasty things you never thought you'd be willing to do. He really brings out the bad girl in you. If you want to give him a taste of oral pleasure before you begin the hand job, disappear under the covers and let your mouth work its magic for a while.

Warm some lubricant between your hands and smother your man's penis and testicles with it until he's slick. Keep your hands moving all over his genitals. Move them over the head of his penis, around the *corona* (the ridge of flesh where the head of the penis meets the shaft), the shaft, the base, the scrotum, the *frenulum* (the strip of flesh on the underside of the penis, where the head meets the shaft), and the perineum. Alternate between strokes and hand squeezes as he lies back to bask in the sensations that are bringing his genitalia to life. Now rub his shaft between your palms like you're starting a fire, then stop quickly and tightly stroke downward.

Starting at the base of his penis, use your well-lubed hands to stroke upward only, one hand immediately after the other, then switch and stroke downward, again one hand quickly followed by the other. Now use the fingers of each hand to form an O (index fingers touching thumbs) and stroke in opposite directions at the same time, so that one ring slides up to the head while the other moves down to the base. As your one hand reaches the top of his shaft, add a twist to the head of the penis; as your other hand reaches the base of his penis, rub your palm against his scrotum. This is kind of a pat-your-head-and-rub-your-stomach move, so don't fret if you can't perform it with total synchronicity; you won't hear any complaining.

When you're ready to make your man climax, change your strokes so they are more predictable and rhythmic, and don't break the rhythm as he nears orgasm. As he gets close, ask him to come on your body, and don't be shy in your request. Tell him you want to feel his hot come land on your skin, you want to see it glisten on your body, and you want to rub it into your flesh. Come on, you can say it. We *dare* you.

You can decide where you want him to ejaculate, or you can let him choose. We'll give you a few suggestions. Lie on your back and have your partner straddle your body so that you can stroke him with your hands and he can come on your belly or breasts. Or, pump his penis between your breasts so he can come on your neck (or your face if you're really game). Arch your back and tell him how hot it feels on your skin as he ejaculates to maximize the mental and visual elements of his orgasm, and flatter him on the amazing amount!

Your man may find it pleasurable to pump himself. He can ejaculate on your vagina or you can get onto your hands and knees and let him come on your bum or back, doggy style. Whatever position you choose and whoever does the work, just remember to react with eager bliss as his ejaculate lands on your body.

A final suggestion . . . but only for the *really* bad girls among us. To rival the antics of those XXX starlets, why

> **Want to let your man pretend you're bathing in his juices but don't really want to do the deed?** While he's inside you, take a handful of body lotion and rub it over your throat, breasts, and belly as he watches, telling him to imagine it's his semen. He'll get a rush, and you'll get moisturized.

not throw your man into the middle of a money shot and let him give you a facial? (Hey, we said it was only for the really bad girls.) Have him stand up as you kneel by his groin and ask him to stroke his cock and watch as he comes in your open mouth. Just like the leading ladies, lick him clean as he finishes. Obviously this isn't for all women. If you feel it's a degrading act, or if your partner makes you feel degraded during the act, simply don't do it; however, the facial is a fantasy for many men, and if your man is worthy of having his fantasies fulfilled, you're the woman to make it happen.

A money shot is a sexy way to dress up an everyday hand job, but don't rely on it exclusively. Although the visual and mental aspects are powerfully erotic, part of the eroticism comes from the novelty and spontaneity. To keep this lube job an effective maintenance sex tool, reserve it for occasional and unexpected use only.

Lube Job #4

●

Grab a Gear—Part I

Have you ever had to work alongside a negative co-worker? You know, one of those people who are chronically irritable. They never smile, never lighten up, and never have anything nice to say about anything or anyone. No doubt someone in the office has commented, "Wow, that Sean guy really has to get laid." We might laugh in response, but we're probably nodding at the same time, for most of us recognize the connection between sex and mood. And cold, hard science can back us up.

Sex, especially when combined with love, has remarkable effects on emotional well-being. The act of sex causes the brain to release a number of neurochemicals, such as endorphins, dopamine, and oxytocin, which create a natural high, no prescription required. When we engage in loving sex, we experience intense feelings of contentment, joy, and lasting affection toward our partner.

Regular sex has other important emotional and psychological benefits. Not only does it reduce stress levels, it also helps us manage stress better as we go through our day. Sex and sexual intimacy can even alleviate depression: endorphins result in a rush of euphoria, and the loving touch of a partner generates feelings of security, acceptance, and happiness. And as Sean's co-workers know, sex is a fun and effective way to reduce irritability.

> **Regular sex improves more than emotional mood; it also increases physical well-being.** Under-the-sheets sessions help improve circulation and lower both cholesterol levels and the risk of heart disease.

The connection between sexual satisfaction and happiness is clear in long-term relationships. All else being equal, couples tend to be happier, both in the relationship and in general, when they are sexually satisfied. This is particularly so for the man in the relationship, since men often have a greater need for sexual desire than women do. That's where maintenance sex comes in. The woman who helps her man stay sexually satisfied is going to have a happier partner than the woman who doesn't. The formula really is that simple.

Jacqueline and Tony, together for ten years, are one couple that has discovered the formula. In fact, Jacqueline has refined it.

"The easiest way to make sure your guy is always satisfied is what I call the Happiness Hand Job," says Jacqueline. "It's a quick fix, nothing more—a tune-up. You can do it almost anywhere. I've been doing them for years in all kinds of places. The first one I ever did was in the car, which I guess is kind of fitting."

As Jacqueline relates, the initiation of the Happiness Hand Job occurred on the morning of Tony's parents' thirty-fifth wedding anniversary: "We were having a surprise anniversary party for his parents in our backyard. It had started out as a small occasion, but soon friends and family were coming in from all over the country and we had all kinds of preparations to make on really short notice. The party was to start at five o'clock, since that's about the time his parents' flight was getting into town. It was in mid-July, and the temperature was over eighty-five degrees, so we had rented this huge outdoor canopy to protect everyone in the backyard from the sun. We were supposed to pick it up at the rental store just before noon, which would've given us plenty of time to set it up, but when we showed up to collect it, they didn't have it in stock."

"I shouldn't have been surprised," says Tony. "Everything seemed to be going wrong. The relatives I couldn't stand had decided to save a buck and crash at our house, so the ones I liked had to stay in hotels. One of my aunts fed our miniature poodle this huge solid chocolate bunny left over from Easter, and it made him sick. We had to rush him to the vet clinic early on a Sunday morning, and that meant a vet bill we could hardly lift. Plus, the kids wouldn't stop crying because they were so worried about the damn dog. Then we couldn't get the barbecue to work. I gave my brother my debit card and had him run out to buy a new one, which he did . . . for seven hundred dollars. I had to pay for it, of course, even though we didn't have that kind of money to spend on a barbecue."

The sweltering heat didn't help, either. "Tony was in the worst mood I'd ever seen him in," says Jacqueline. "Though nobody could blame him. It was a stressful day, and nothing was going our way. What should've been a fun time was just miserable. Some of his relatives were really demanding and expected us to wait on them hand and foot, in addition to taking care of all the prep for the party. The heat was a killer, too. It made everybody extra testy, just because they felt so uncomfortable. Tony can't handle the heat at all, so he was particularly grumpy. When they told us the canopy wasn't available even though we'd prepaid and booked it, I thought Tony was going to completely lose it."

> ✳ **Many studies have demonstrated the link between sex and longevity. The more time you spend doing it, the more time you'll have to spend.**

"I don't know when I've been so pissed off," explains Tony. "I can still remember how angry I was. I was just miserable. I wanted to go back and tell everybody the party was off and they could . . . you know what."

So, with the sun beating down on them in the car and the air conditioning blasting out on high, Jacqueline and Tony began to drive around the city, hitting all the rental shops in their desperate search for an outdoor canopy. Unfortunately, mid-July was prime wedding season, and the search was proving to be fruitless.

"Every store we went into just laughed at us," says Jacqueline. "Everybody in the state was getting married that weekend, so there weren't any outdoor canopies left to rent. It was horrible. We were hot, irritable as hell, and the day seemed to be getting worse by the second. After we left the last rental store empty handed, Tony slapped the steering wheel in anger. I felt terrible for him. It should've been a happy day, but it was just frustrating."

Jacqueline knew something had to be done if the day was to be salvaged.

"I said, 'Tony, you need to calm down.' He said, 'Jackie, I need to get laid.'"

To Jacqueline's amazement, they proceeded to have an argument about, of all things, sex.

"I couldn't believe it. We had a houseful of people waiting for us, all kinds of errands still to run, and there we were, parked in front of the rental store, having a fight about how long it'd been since we'd had sex. I told Tony we had more important things to worry about at that moment, but he wasn't listening to me."

"I was so mad that I was just venting all my frustrations," says Tony. "I was letting it all out. I thought about the last few nights that I'd tried to initiate sex but had been turned down for whatever reason. I was more pissed off about that than I was about not finding a big umbrella. I didn't care who got heatstroke, I really needed some relief."

"We didn't have time to go home and have sex," explains Jacqueline. "Anyway, we had a houseful of guests wandering around, so there was no privacy. But I knew I had to do something, or the whole day was going to be ruined. Tony's attitude really needed adjusting. Fast."

Jacqueline thought. She remembered the plastic bag lying on the backseat, the one from the drugstore, and reached around to grab it. Then she instructed Tony to drive around the back of the rental store and to park in a secluded spot behind a dumpster. Sensing something good was in the air, he followed orders no-questions-asked.

"Jackie started rummaging through the bag," recalls Tony. "She pulled out a bottle of her face cleanser and a pack of baby wipes, then told me to unzip my pants. I had them open before she finished the sentence. I felt like I had won the lottery."

> Sex can also improve overall fitness. A half hour of vigorous mattress maneuvers can burn two hundred calories and can get that heart rate up. So walk right by the treadmill and work up a sweat with your partner instead.

"That was the first Happiness Hand Job I'd ever given," says Jacqueline. "Even though it was improvised, it was probably one of the best. Although there have been some runners-up in the years since."

"It took about three minutes, but it was three minutes that changed my whole mood. It was like somebody had released the pressure, and my frustration just dissolved into the air. I felt almost giddy from the relief, and all the things that were upsetting me started to seem funny. I was way more relaxed, and I got my sense of humor back. I'm not exaggerating when I say it saved the day."

Needless to say, the anniversary party was enjoyed by all . . . even *sans* canopy. But there's no reason you have to wait for a special occasion to treat your partner to a Happiness Hand Job. Chances are, this quick fix could be a valuable part of regular maintenance. It's a fast, convenient, and exciting way to pleasure a man, and it has positive effects on both his physical and emotional well-being.

While a hand job can be performed in many locales, from your private bedroom to a public bathroom, the car is a great place to start exploring *terra incognita*. By parking in a secluded area, you have the best of both worlds: You get the thrill of doing it in different public spaces, yet you have the safety of your own secured space. Plus, being sexually serviced in the car is one of a man's greatest fantasies. It lets him toy with the idea of indecency, which in itself can boost a man's libido. Yet when it comes to car sex, don't let your excitement compromise your common sense. Lock your doors and choose a spot where there's no chance of passersby, be they innocent, dangerous, or on patrol.

> **Want to fight the flu?** You can do more than pop echinacea and wash your hands; sex also helps to strengthen the immune system. And if one of those nasty cold bugs does slip through, sex can still help; the adrenaline released during the act is a natural antihistamine.

To make sure you're always prepared to perform an on-the-go lube job, keep a stash of lubricant either in your glove box or in your purse. A travel pack of baby wipes or at least a box of strong tissue is convenient for cleanup. If you prefer, there are postcoital wipes available at sex shops and online that are nice and thick for janitorial purposes.

You'll probably be most at ease performing your first few in-car hand jobs in totally secluded areas; however, your courage may grow with time and experience. As far as car sex goes, hand jobs are relatively low risk. You're not in an overly compromising position, and if some nosy passerby does peek through the windshield, you can quickly put that empty fast-food bag over your partner's lap to cover your tracks.

After the car is safely in park, tell your man to put his seat back a little and prepare to be serviced. Unfasten his pants and push them and his underwear down so that he can sit back and enjoy the process of having you expose him like this. If he wants, let him undo his own pants so he has a sense of power; he may want to pretend he's paying for the encounter!

As always, warm the lube between your hands before you apply it to your partner's penis. Scratch his pubic hair with your fingertips, fondle his testicles, then hook your fingers into the claw position to pull up on his penis. When he's hard, you can begin to stroke him in a way that pleases him. Tell him to lean back in his seat, put his hands on the wheel, and brace himself for impact as you bring him to orgasm.

This lube job has three things going for it. First, there's the spontaneity. You're seizing the moment and gratifying

> There's maintenance sex, and then there's medicinal sex. The next time you strain that tennis elbow, reach for your partner instead of the ibuprofen. Having sex releases endorphins that offer natural pain relief.

your man when he needs it most, and he won't be expecting that. Men are accustomed to waiting . . . and waiting . . . and waiting for sexual release, but this lube job brings him to the front of the line. Second, there's the novelty of a sexual experience in the car. Since the vast majority of sexual activity happens in our bedrooms, it's an intensely erotic—and taboo—experience to feel sexual pleasure beyond the bedroom walls. Third, sitting upright may be a somewhat uncommon position for your man to receive a hand job, with lying or standing being more familiar.

Put these three elements together, and you've found a fantastic, on-the-fly way to perform maintenance sex. You've also discovered a simple yet fun way to add a few sparks to your sex life. But perhaps most important, you've realized the connection between sexual satisfaction and emotional well-being, and you've taken the time to ensure that the man you love has plenty of both. And why not? The happier you make him, the happier he will make you, and the more fulfilling your relationship will be.

Lube Job #5

●

Backseat Driver

Nobody seems to take the poor hand job seriously. There are books on fellatio, intercourse, anal sex, etc., but what about the traditional tug many of us first pleasured our partners with? It seems it's been banished to the outskirts of a couple's sex life, only occasionally called out of exile to perform ultra-utilitarian, get-it-done duty sex. Yet as the chapters in this section have shown, it takes only good technique and creativity to make this faithful standby a new favorite. It's time the ancient palm practice of manual manipulation was revived to challenge modern woman to get her hands dirty once in a while.

The truth is, the hand job is a versatile yet simple way to make the most mundane maintenance sex session into a memorable sexual experience. Using your hands has definite advantages: you can manipulate your man's genitals in precise ways; you can apply very different degrees of pressure, rhythm, and sensation; and you can do it quickly, easily, and discreetly in all types of locations. A hand job is only bland if you let it be, and we hope these chapters have inspired you to revisit and revamp this maintenance must-have.

> To convince your man that you're enthusiastic about satisfying him, make the first move and initiate maintenance sex more often. Why wait for him to beg? Beat him to the punch and show him that his pleasure is your priority.

Another advantage of the hand job is that you can see exactly what you're doing, and, with a little direction from your partner, you can use your viewpoint to learn a lot about his body and what pleasures him. In this lube job, he is the quintessential backseat driver, and you're at the wheel as he guides you on a journey of sexual exploration.

The next time you're uninterested in sex but your man is making the moves, have him lie back on the bed, naked and relaxed, with his hands leisurely behind his head. He's a passenger on this ride, albeit the one holding the map, so he can kick back while you play chauffeur. Have some personal lubricant close by. Straddle his body backward, so that he's looking up at your back and you're looking at his feet. Flash him a smile over your shoulder, and tell him that you want to please him *exactly* the way he wants to be pleased, that you want to learn what turns him on, and you want him to teach you.

Warm some lube between your hands, but before you

apply it to his genitals, ask him where he'd like to feel it first. Does he want it on his balls first? The shaft of his penis? The head? Now ask how he'd like you to apply it. With long strokes? With your fingers, like you're rubbing lotion into his skin? A combination?

After he's slicked up, ask him to lead you through this hand job. He should direct you where and how to stroke and for how long; where to squeeze or twist, when, and at what pressure and pace. Make sure he keeps talking throughout, even if you're prompting him every few moments by saying "Do you like it like this or like that? Should I stroke harder or softer? Faster or slower? Would a twist feel good now? How does it feel when I put pressure here or tickle there? Do you want me to stroke you to orgasm, or do you want to let it build longer?"

> **Cat got your tongue? Pillow talk is one thing, but talking *during* sex is another. Some love it, others find it downright distracting. Talk to your partner about what you want to hear in the throes of passion. At the very least, an "I love you" or "That feels wonderful" shouldn't be too verbose.**

Be sure to keep your man talking as his orgasm mounts and even as he comes. Tell him you want to learn all you can about what he's feeling at every point and that you want to watch his cock and see how it changes when something feels good. Does it twitch or swell? Do his balls get tighter or raise up to his penis? What does it look like when he's coming? Lean over to get a closer look, in the process giving your man a delicious view of your backside as he ejaculates.

When you show this intense level of interest in your man's genitals and pleasure, you appeal to his sexual ego and increase his arousal. Unfortunately, men are often all too aware of when they're receiving pure maintenance sex, which can't be much of a turn-on. Would you feel comfortable exposing your sexual needs or seeking satisfaction from your man if he seemed distracted while he was pleasuring you?

"I always knew when my girlfriend was doing it for maintenance," says Trevor, twenty-seven. "She'd start out okay, but a couple minutes into it and she'd tune out. The stroking wouldn't be rhythmic, and her face would be wrinkled up because she was thinking about something else. I'd close my eyes and not look at her. I'd just live out some fantasy and try to get what I could out of it. No, it wasn't a really good time, and it was hard to stay aroused at times. The orgasm just took the pressure off. It wasn't ever great."

Even if you're the silent type during sex, *always* speak up when you want to guide your man to better pleasure you. And make sure he knows the flow of communication goes both ways.

Despite the importance of tuning in to your man's pleasure, it's sometimes difficult for a woman to fake sincere interest and enthusiasm when performing maintenance sex, especially if she's tired, irritated, or has other things on her mind. If that's the case with you, this lube job is ideal. By following his directions, you focus on him only. And each time you ask him a question about his body—Does it feel good when I do this?—you show him how important his pleasure is to you. Chances are, his gratitude will rouse your affection for him, and your mood will improve. At the very least, any guilt you have about not satisfying his sexual cravings will be alleviated.

Letting your man be the backseat driver is one more way the simple but versatile hand job can outperform the competition when it comes to maintenance sex.

Part Two

Fellatio

Lube Job #6

●

You've Got Male

> I've been thinking about you all day . . .
about how you taste and what I'd like to do
to you.

>> *What would you like to do to me?*

> I'd like to kneel down in front of you and
put my hands on your hips. I'd like to swallow that hard, gorgeous cock of yours and
suck and lick and suck until I can feel the
veins in the shaft swell and throb under my
tongue and I know you're ready to come.

>> *And then what would you do?*

> I'd swallow as much of your cock as I could,
letting the swollen head stay deep in my
throat until I hear you moan and I feel the
hot come jet out of you and burn down my
throat . . .

>> *I'll be home in fifteen minutes!*

> I'll put the baby down for her nap!

Whew! Although parts of the above conversation might read like an anonymous exchange in the murky backwaters of an online chat room, it's no such thing. In reality, the above dialogue is the cheeky electronic sex script between two loving, longtime partners.

Tyler and Jenn were high school sweethearts who have managed to dodge the statistics by recently celebrating their fifteenth wedding anniversary. Married young (Jenn was only eighteen when they exchanged I do's), their relationship and their marriage has had to grow and change and mature just as they themselves have had to. Like all long-term couples, their sex life has gone through more ups and downs than they can remember. Like all successful and happy long-term couples, they've managed to ride the rises and falls like kids on a roller coaster: they throw their arms up and shriek with joy when things are fun and hold on tight when things are scary.

Unlike many couples, Tyler and Jenn were married almost twelve years before they had their first child. Tyler took over the family transportation business right out of high school, and Jenn pursued a career as a teacher before becoming the principal of an elementary school. A self-described power couple, they spent years earning and traveling before finally deciding it was time for baby-makes-three status.

As all new parents quickly discover, *baby* starts with a capital B. For Boss. No longer could Tyler and Jenn actually finish a meal without a wail from the nursery. No longer could they watch a movie without having to hit pause for a diaper change. No longer could they enjoy a cuddle on the couch without having to stop halfway for

Jenn to haul out the breast pump and dutifully produce. No longer did Tyler come first. Now in her early thirties, Jenn was all about the baby. Now, maintenance sex, which had always been a part of their sex life, was more important than ever.

> ☼ **THE BREAST-FEEDING BABY BLUES**
> **The hormones released by breast feeding can lead to vaginal dryness in many women. If this uncomfortable side effect of good mothering is preventing you from getting back in the sexual saddle, ask your man to stimulate you with a well-lubed finger before you automatically pass on the pleasures of intercourse.**

Having chosen to stay home with their new daughter, Jenn soon found herself feeling insecure for the first time in her marriage. For years, she had left for work, dressed smartly in her business suit and pumps, at the same time in the morning as Tyler. Now, she kissed him good-bye at the door in her bathrobe, the same one she was often in when she welcomed him at the door that evening.

She admitted it. She was getting the frumps. Worse, Jenn felt as though motherhood was replacing her womanhood and that in the process she was losing her sexuality. Maybe it was somewhere in the backseat of her car under the crushed box of teething biscuits. Maybe it was hiding under the top drawer of her dresser under her extra stash of breast-feeding pads. Or maybe it had sprinted away at the sight of the heavy black bags of babyhood that now hung under her eyes. Wherever it was, it was moving further away from ever being found, and Jenn knew she had to do something to reclaim it. She knew that of all the changes her marriage had survived over the years, this would be the biggest and the most rewarding.

Strangely enough, the change came about by electronic accident. One morning, after Tyler had left for work, Jenn was checking her e-mail on her home computer. As she shuffled her slippers on the floor underneath the desk and slurped her fourth cup of coffee, she received an e-mail that she thought was from Tyler's new address at work.

When she opened the e-mail, it became clear to Jenn that this message had originated from neither her husband's computer nor from his mind. The e-mail was of the "longer, harder, thicker" variety and was accompanied by a short but provocative testimonial from one of the questionable product's very satisfied customers. Despite herself, Jenn found herself reading the explicit nature of the testimonial and becoming almost . . . aroused!

Feeling suddenly very inspired—and frisky—she fired off a flirtatious e-mail to Tyler at work. Instead of responding hours later as he usually did (for example, when she e-mailed to share news of the baby's noteworthy bowel movements), he replied almost immediately.

To Jenn's surprise and delight, Tyler's e-mail had upped the ante and was even racier than hers. Jenn knew immediately that she had tapped into a deep well of erotic potential. She also realized that her husband's almost too-eager response to her flirtatiousness was evidence that he was not receiving the level of sexual attention he needed. And so began an electric affair of sorts between a husband and wife. Gradually, the innocent "I'd love to kiss you right nows" turned into hardcore "I'd love to taste your come in my mouth right nows." Happily, the baby's gastrointestinal status was no longer discussed online.

Despite the flurry of regular and increasingly raunchy e-mail Jenn began to exchange with her husband, she admits that she often participated in this sexy correspondence for the express purpose of keeping Tyler's sexual interest focused on her. Instead of succumbing to the frumps—the emotional, physical, and sexual frumps—she would tease him with an e-mail describing the sexy bra she was sporting. When he came home, she would of course

> **Fight the frumps with fitness. Exercise not only improves our mood by releasing endorphins, it also increases blood flow to the genitals, which leads to arousal. Don't neglect your nether regions during your workout; Kegel exercises strengthen the vagina and make it better able to grasp the penis during sex.**

be wearing it, regardless of whether she was really in the mood to lift and separate.

What followed may have been maintenance sex, but nobody peering through the bedroom window could have guessed it. Not only did Jenn's efforts ensure that her husband remained interested in her and was sexually satisfied, but they also inspired her to keep her thoughts and actions sexual. As maintenance sex so often does, it helped keep the embers of her own sexuality going until she had learned to merge motherhood and womanhood, and could again watch her flames shoot high into the sky.

Let's take this opportunity to tap into Jenn's well of electronic eroticism. It's a timely method of foreplay, and most men are more than techno-savvy enough to play along. When they're not checking their odometers, it seems that many men are busy checking their e-mail. Most of us are regular users of a computer, and it's likely that sometime during your evening you'll find yourself staring at the screen, working, surfing, or checking those endless e-mail messages. And that's a good thing, since that's exactly where you need to be to get this strictly maintenance lube job done.

Before you perform this lube job, and if circumstances permit, send your partner a few provocative e-mail messages during his workday. Don't be bashful. If you're at home, describe the sexy panties you're wearing (lie if you must), or tell him about the hot and steamy bath you just took, hot and steamy because of the things you were thinking about doing with him. If you're at work, describe how you're sitting at your desk with your legs crossed to stimulate yourself while you think about all the things you want to do to his body tonight. Say the things you know will turn him on and let him stare at the clock, willing it to release him so he can come home to the delight that so eagerly awaits him. You can even create alter ego e-mail accounts for each of you, reserved exclusively for the exchange of these very personal messages.

If he doesn't have access to e-mail (or if you don't want to risk the boss intercepting this naughty non-business-related correspondence), slip a sexy note into your man's pocket before he leaves for work, or leave a suggestive message in his lunch box or briefcase instead. You can even text-message a love note on his cell phone.

Regardless of how they're delivered, these messages will make your man feel genuinely wanted. Just as women long to feel reassured and cherished, men thrive when they feel needed and desired. For men, the feeling of being needed by a woman often leads to or enhances his sexual feelings for her. Use this instinctual connection to your advantage. Flatter him, let him know you need and want him, and let his desire for you build throughout the day. By the time he gets home, he'll be ready to burst forth at your touch.

When you and your partner are at last at home together and you're working on the computer, pull up a blank screen and discreetly compose a raunchy message to your partner. Again, don't be shy. Type something like:

```
I've been thinking about you all day...
about taking your cock in my mouth and suck-
ing it until you burst in my mouth. I've been
imagining your cock pressed against my lips,
thinking about how wonderful and hard it
feels when you push it past my lips and it
sinks into my mouth. I can't wait to stroke
```

and suck until I feel you erupt down my
throat. I can't wait to feel your hips rock
back and forth and your hands clutch my hair
as you come hard and fast. . . .

Remember, you're trying to get him aroused quickly, so
don't write about rose petals and your feelings. Use the
power of dirty talk to turn him on. Write about how desperately you want to pleasure him and about how good the
rush of his orgasm will feel.

Next, casually call your partner into the room and nonchalantly ask him to read the message as if it were a frivolous forward from a mutual friend. As your man's mind
registers the content and he realizes that he's the lucky recipient, spin around in your chair and offer him a wicked
grin. Reach out to fondle his genitals (over his pants) to

> Writer's block? Since you're on the computer anyway, scan a free online erotica
> site to increase your sexual vocabulary. Just
> make sure you do it on your own time and with
> your own PC, not the company's!

arouse him. When you feel his bulge, unzip his pants and
push them and his underwear down to just below his
bum. You just need access to his genitals, you don't need
him completely undressed. Such is the convenience of a
quickie.

Spend a moment in blatant admiration of your partner's manhood before asking him to spread his legs and relax. As he does, slip down onto your knees in front of him: if you want, you can unfasten your top few buttons to allow him a delicious bird's-eye view of your sexy bra-clad breasts. Gently fondle your man's perineum and massage his testicles until he is at least semi-erect. Hook your arms behind his bum as if locking yourself to him, and bring your mouth close to his groin. Blow hot breath onto his genitals and moan to show how anxious you are to take him in your mouth.

If he's soft or if you want to torture him a bit longer, begin with some teasing tongue moves before putting his penis in your mouth. Nuzzle your face into his perineum and lick it. Use the tip of your tongue to trace around his genitals. Starting at his perineum, circle his scrotum and then drag your tongue over his testicles to the base of his penis. Circle the base of his penis, then flatten your tongue and lick the underside of his shaft from the base to the frenulum. Because the frenulum is an exceptionally sensitive area, don't use too much pressure the first time you stimulate it. Point your tongue again, flick the tip against the frenulum, and then trace a complete circle under the ridge of the glans. Finally, flatten your tongue once again and lick the head of his penis like an ice-cream cone. This exquisite process should make his penis erect, or at least semi-erect, in record time.

When your partner is hard enough for fellatio, slowly take about half the length of his penis into your mouth. At the same time, clutch and caress his buttocks to make what you're doing even naughtier and to increase his arousal. Suck and lick his penis very gently for a few moments, hands free, kneading his buttocks and rocking his groin into your mouth.

When you're ready to rev his engine harder, allow just the head of his penis to pass through your lips and then close your lips tightly around the shaft. Treat the head of his penis to a good tongue-lashing while it's inside your mouth: swirl your tongue around it, circle the ridge, and then slide the bumpy underside of your tongue over top of the glans to vary the sensations he is experiencing inside the wonderful warm wetness of your mouth.

Now take as much of his shaft as you can into your mouth, making a show of just how big he really is. Suck firmly as you slide your mouth up and off his penis, letting your lips pop over the ridge of the glans. To begin the downstroke, purse your lips and press them against the glans, offering slight resistance before allowing the head of his penis to break through the barrier of your lips and sink into the depths of your mouth. Stroke his penis a few times in this way and be sure that your moans and move-ments express how wonderful he tastes.

Stop stroking for a moment and direct your partner to hold his penis with one hand, at the base, and to push your mouth onto it. This will give him a powerful and gritty sense of sexual control that will add to the "dirtiness" of what you're doing. Let him be as forceful as both your comfort zones allow.

When you want to bring your man to orgasm, hold his penis at the base with one hand while with the other hand you squeeze and tug his testicles, gently pulling them away from his body. To begin a momentum-building rhythm with good pressure around his penis, form a ring with your fingers and tightly stroke his shaft while simultaneously performing fellatio: hold your hand close to your mouth and continue to suck his penis while you milk and squeeze it with your fingers. Adopt the pace, pressure, and rhythm you know will make him come, and let him ejaculate in your mouth.

Spit or swallow? Check the menu before deciding. Many women claim that a man's semen tastes different after he's eaten certain types of foods. Dairy products, meat, and alcohol are generally thought to worsen taste, while fruit and vegetables are believed to improve it.

Whether you swallow your partner's semen depends on you: if you're reluctant to, it's no matter. Simply have a tissue nearby to strategically rid yourself of the evidence. Whatever you do, *don't* make a spectacle of this. The last thing your man wants to think is that you find his body or his juices in any way distasteful. If you have to spit, you can always tell him there was just too much to swallow. Many men see the volume of their ejaculate as an indication of their virility, so this may be one way to spare his feelings and flatter him at the same time. Be discreet and respectful, while still honoring what you are willing to do and not do.

Of course, there is a wealth of fellatio techniques available in this handbook (as well as on the Internet and on video), and while skill is important and helpful, a good knowledge of what turns your particular man on is far more valuable. It isn't necessary to concern yourself with using a wide variety of professional porn-sanctioned techniques during a lube job. In the end, these maintenance quickies work because, from your partner's perspective, they are completely spontaneous and perhaps somewhat out of character for you. His spike of arousal and quick climax don't come from flawless textbook maneuvers; they come from the sheer thrill of the experience itself.

> **What an eyeful! When you're performing fellatio on your man, glance up at him and maintain eye contact while you suck. It's a turn-on for many guys.**

Now that you've satisfied your partner, send him into the kitchen on shaky legs to prepare a postfellatio snack while you power-down the computer. Working through all that e-mail may have worked up your appetites.

Lube Job #7

●

The Hot-Oil Change

Women don't always understand the male preoccupation with The Penis. Is it too small? Too skinny? Too crooked? Do women find it attractive? It seems as if men are far more concerned with these penile issues than women are. Yet the fairer sex can certainly sympathize, for in this age of airbrushed beauty, surgical nips and tucks, suctions, injections, lifts, and enlargements, women suffer from a constant and brutal onslaught of culturally imposed and completely impossible standards of bodily perfection and eternal youth.

Popular culture and its conniving twin sister, advertising, send out a common message to both sexes—your body just isn't good enough. The insecurities these calculating beasts spread too often spill into our intimate relationships, causing problems where before there were none or few. So where is one to find shelter from a storm of heartless criticism? In the arms of one's beloved, of course. Now more than ever it is vital to the health and happiness of a couple's sex life for each partner to know that his or her body is desirable to the other. Sincere sexual flattery is essential to maintaining a good love life.

Just days before starting this chapter, Don and I were channel-surfing when a major beauty pageant, in the full throes of the swimsuit competition no less, flashed across the screen. Don had the remote control, and instead of slowing to watch he passed by without missing a beat, saying "Those plastics have nothing on my wife." I thought to myself, What woman wouldn't want a husband like this? Snuggling closer to him on the couch, I told him how much his reaction meant to me: how it made me feel loved, confident, and very, very, frisky. Most important, it made me feel protected from the weapons of mass demoralization that our culture is constantly firing at women.

Don's response to my expression of gratitude was an enlightening one, and it actually provided the impetus for this lube job. As it turns out, his female-friendly reaction to the beauty pageant was in part caused by an incident that had happened a few years earlier. He reminded me of a television program we had seen, and although it took a while for me to remember it, it was obviously still front and center in his memory.

The program was a documentary of sorts, on penises. Human penises of every size, shape, color, slant, length, width, and appearance were shown, some hanging down, some standing up at full attention, a few somewhere in between. According to Don, I responded by watching for a few minutes with mild amusement and then turning off the television and gushing about how perfect his manhood was, how it was more desirable than any I had seen on the television, and how I felt so lucky to be married to such a fine specimen. Little did I know it, but my lighthearted penis praise had actually had a profound and lasting impact on our marriage. While this may seem absurd at first, if you really think about it, there was great wisdom in my approach.

We all know that the better you make someone feel about himself or herself, the better that person will feel about you. In friendship, we're all drawn to people who build us up, and we avoid those who tear us down. That simple logic extends to our intimate relationships. No one in the world has more power over another person's sexual confidence than does that person's spouse or intimate partner. By consciously deciding to shield each other from the sexual insecurities that can so ruthlessly invade our psyches, a couple builds a fortress around their sexual relationship that nothing can break through. They also reaffirm the love, devotion, and admiration they have for each other in other areas of their life together. Praise is power.

> **It is better to give than to receive.**
> **Giving compliments to our partners can remind us of their positive traits and increase our sexual desire for them.**

Of course, the real issue isn't whose penis is straighter or better looking (or whose breasts are fuller or nicer). The real issue is good stewardship. We give more than just our bodies to our partners. We give our hearts and souls, too, and when those aren't handled with as much love and care as our bodies, the relationship suffers. We women thrive in relationships when men take the time to compliment us, whether it's to tell us that we look sexy in a dress, that we're smart, that our skin feels soft, or that our breasts are beautiful. These compliments not only give us personal confidence, they also strengthen our feelings of commitment and love for our mate.

Yet there is something of a double standard when it comes to flattering men. For some reason, there isn't the same tendency to compliment a man as there is a woman, even though—ask any man—a sincere compliment can make the sun shine brighter on even the darkest days. Quite often, a woman will make a mental note of how handsome or sexy her man looks but will nonetheless fail to vocalize the compliment, perhaps assuming that such praise isn't as important to him as it is to her.

Unfortunately, the failure to flatter our men isn't always an innocent oversight. Nicole, a twenty-eight-year-old wife and mother of two, came to think of complimenting her husband as a weakness. Regardless of how good he looked or how hard he tried to please her, she withheld praise, fearing that it might go to his head. And praise isn't all that she withheld. Sex soon followed.

"I used to throw the compliments around like they were going out of style," Nicole says. "We were in love, in the honeymoon phase, and I was forever telling him how sweet he was."

So what caused the change?

"Peer pressure," admits Nicole. "Pure and simple. It's embarrassing now, but I started hanging around some women who all bitched nonstop about the men in their lives, and before I knew it, I began thinking like them. I was no better than an impressionable teenager: they'd slam their ex-husbands or boyfriends, and I'd be right alongside them, joining in. At first it was just talk, but then it started to take root, and my whole attitude deteriorated."

"It was like Jekyll and Hyde," says Nicole's husband, Marty. "For the first five or six years of our marriage she was adorable and always said the nicest things. Then we seemed to hit a brick wall. I call that brick wall 'Mommy's new friends.'"

Mommy's new friends were a group of women Nicole met when her younger daughter began preschool. These moms seemed harmless enough at first, so Nicole was happy when they invited her to their regular Friday movie night, which was held at one of the single mom's houses. For the first several Fridays, the outings were a welcome break from her routine, and she looked forward to the camaraderie of having girlfriends around for the first time since her college days. The girl talk, laughter, and common interests reminded her of her single days, before the husband and kids.

"Most of the moms were divorced or never married, so the girl talk was different than with my happily married friends," says Nicole. "I had a sense of independence and freedom that reminded me of when I was single. Don't get me wrong, they were terrific mothers to their kids, but because most of them weren't tied down to a man, the conversation seemed a lot more colorful—youthful—to me, and I felt more youthful just being there."

But gradually, the girl talk gave way to unadulterated man bashing. One woman told of how her ex-husband cheated on her, while another revealed the sordid details of her own string of infidelities. An unhappy wife told of how her current husband spent more time playing with his video games than he did with his own kids. Yet another woman complained that her live-in boyfriend was more concerned about his ex-wife than he was about her, even though they were planning to marry and he had been divorced for years.

When Nicole sheepishly admitted that her husband was both faithful and very involved in their children's lives, her comments were met with derision and ridicule: "Whenever I said I was happy in my marriage, they'd all laugh and treat me like I was a naive schoolgirl. They'd say the ax would fall any day and I'd realize all men are alike. I managed to ignore them for a while and just told myself they were bitter, but it was like they managed to plant this tiny seed of doubt that really stuck."

> **Peer pressure can be positive too.**
> **Surround yourself with happy, fulfilled, and well-balanced people to reap the benefits of positive peer pressure.**

Soon, the tiny seed of doubt began to grow into a big change of behavior. "When I'd get home after a Friday movie night, I'd always walk through the door with a chip on my shoulder," admits Nicole. "If Marty had fallen asleep on the couch waiting for me, I'd think, What an asshole! Those women are right. If he'd cleaned the house and was waiting up for me, I'd think, What a suck-up. What's he trying to hide?"

And of course, their sex life began to be affected as Nicole's attitude toward sex changed, too. "Sex was always a hot topic of conversation on these movie nights. My friends were always saying how they weren't put on the planet just to satisfy some man's needs, and I wondered if that's what I was doing. Marty's always had a really strong sex drive, and I often did it when I wasn't in the mood, just to satisfy him. But now I had the idea that satisfying him was beneath me. If he hinted that he wanted sex, it just made me angry."

Over the weeks, the situation grew worse. Nicole became increasing intolerant, critical, and unloving. Marty withdrew to the basement and began to play solitaire on the computer instead of engaging with his family. "I didn't want to be anywhere near her," says Marty. "Bad vibes were all I got from her and lots of them. I wouldn't be surprised if we went two months without her saying a single kind word to me. Sex was out of the question. Unless Nicole was *really* in the mood, I didn't stand a chance. It didn't matter how affectionate I was to her; she wouldn't reciprocate in a sexual way, although she knew full well what I wanted."

"Marty would avoid me all night, then crawl into bed at midnight and start reaching for me," says Nicole. "I knew what he wanted, but I deliberately withheld it. Looking back, it was very cruel, but at the time it seemed totally justified. I thought, What am I, your sex slave? I'd never thought about maintenance sex like that in the past, but I was just focused on *my* needs, not his. The more I knew he needed me, the bigger the chip on my shoulder got."

This simmering situation finally erupted one night in the most disturbing way. Nicole came home from a Friday movie night to find Marty asleep on the downstairs couch, the place where he now spent most of his time and sometimes even spent the night. Beside the couch, the screen saver on the computer screen flickered. For some reason, Nicole reached out and clicked the mouse. Her jaw dropped.

"Porn, porn, porn," says Nicole. "It was the home page of a porn site, with a dozen women in really graphic close-ups and a flashing 'Join Now' banner scrolling across the screen. It was ridiculous. In a split second, my married life became a pathetic cliché. There I was, out with the girls while my husband was hiding in the basement, surfing porn on the Web. I remember kicking the computer desk as hard as I could to wake him up. Marty jumped up off the couch, and when he saw that I had discovered his dirty little secret, he just stared at me. He didn't apologize or explain or anything. It was like he didn't even care."

"It's not that I didn't care," Marty explains, "I just wasn't up for the fight. I knew it was the ammunition she was waiting for. It was the proof that her girlfriends were right and that I was an asshole, just like every other man out there."

"I turned around and marched out of the house," says Nicole. "I headed right back to my friend's house. The other women were still there, and I started crying and yelling, telling them what had happened."

Mommy's new friends reacted exactly as Nicole anticipated they would. They told her that Marty was a pervert, a sexual deviant, and that he shouldn't even be around his own kids. They told her that she was too good for him and that he obviously wasn't attracted to her anymore, so she might as well leave. They told her that if she had any self-respect she would divorce him; otherwise she was nothing more than a weak and foolish woman. They told her to pack up his clothes, kick him out, and not let him see his kids until he'd received therapy. They told her she deserved better than a sex-addict husband.

"I think that in my heart I knew it was wrong," says Nicole, "but the whole mess seemed to take on a life of its own. It had its own momentum. I went back home, but I banished Marty to the basement. I even implied that he shouldn't be left alone with his kids—that's the part I still can't forgive myself for. There are some things you say that you can't take back; some things change the way you feel about yourself forever, and that was one of them. I still feel overwhelming shame for that. I don't think I could've forgiven Marty if he had said those things about me, so I don't know how he's found it in his heart to forgive me. I still can't believe that I let myself lose so much perspective."

It was during this time—with Marty sequestered in the basement and Nicole ruling with a heavy hand—that an unexpected houseguest added herself to the volatile situation. Nicole's mother showed up on their doorstep, unannounced and completely oblivious to the hostile territory she was entering. She had been waiting to see a medical specialist in town for some time and had been offered an appointment after a last-minute cancellation.

Nicole told her mother everything that had happened, but her mother's reaction wasn't what she had expected. Instead of automatically joining in her anti-Marty tirade, Nicole's mother asked a question that took her daughter completely off guard.

"My mom asked, 'Why is he looking at pornography? Aren't you putting out?' Honestly, I didn't even know my mom knew the phrase 'putting out.' But her question hit a sore spot, and I started ranting about how it didn't matter whether or not I was putting out, he shouldn't be hiding in the basement looking at porn on the computer."

But Nicole's mother was unmoved by her rant and continued to question her about what was going on in the marriage.

"I was so mad at her. I told her that she was my mother, and that if anyone should stick up for me, it was her. I told her about how my friends had stuck up for me and what they had said, and she started shaking her head. Maybe it was a sixth sense or maybe it was just mother's instinct, but my mom was instantly suspicious of my new friends. She kept saying 'Misery loves company.'"

Unlike Nicole's newfound friends, her mother was clearly invested in her happiness and genuinely wanted what was best for her. She sat Nicole down and calmly assessed the situation. The images on the computer were soft-core pornography. There was nothing violent, under-age, or otherwise overtly disturbing. There were only pictures—no online chatting or friends—and nothing had been actually saved onto the computer. Basically, Marty was looking at a few dirty pictures, and, according to Nicole's mother, that wasn't a hanging offense.

"I told my mom that men shouldn't be looking at porn online and that Marty was a sex addict. She laughed in my face and said that if looking at pictures of naked women made a man a sex addict, then my father and grandfather were sex addicts too. She told me my dad used to have a subscription to a skin magazine and my grandpa had a col-lection of dirty playing cards. I couldn't believe the way my mom was talking since she was always very conservative when it came to sex. She obviously knew I needed the hard line to get my thinking back on track."

> **Pornographic images reach back to antiquity, gracing walls and vases, and also have found expression in sculpture. It seems our ancestors felt the same desire to sneak a peek, but they just couldn't download stone pictures!**

Nicole's mom was even so bold as to ask about her daughter's sex life, and she was unimpressed when she learned her daughter was withholding sex.

"My mom said, 'What do you expect, Nicole? If you turn the taps off upstairs, he's going to go downstairs for a drink.' I hated her for being so rational and especially for being so *right*. I had turned the taps off, and I wasn't even sure why. The more I thought about how I'd been treating him, the more I started to panic. The haze started to clear, and I realized how miserable I'd been to him. He'd been trying so hard to please me, but I'd been mean to him for absolutely no reason. I was terrified there was no going back. My mom said, 'Start being nice. It's that simple.'"

So Nicole started being nice. When Friday came along, she stayed home and spent the movie night with her husband. "I rented his favorite movie, put extra butter on the popcorn, and showered him with praise as well as apologies. My mom was right, it was that simple. In one night I started to undo a lot of the damage that I had done. I told Marty how foolish I'd been acting, how I'd gotten caught up in everything, and how I'd never take him for granted again. I especially told him how wonderful he was and how lucky I was to have a man like him. I went through all his wonderful qualities, from good provider to fantastic lover. His eyes just lit up, and I felt like I could burst into tears. He was like a little boy who'd been ignored for a long time, and now somebody was being kind to him."

"And she put out," adds Marty. "Really well, if I remember clearly. I have one hell of a mother-in-law."

Some of us will never lose as much perspective as Nicole did, and some may have a keener sense of when they're being led down a dark path. Still, we can all empathize with being swept up in something, and, for any number of reasons, we're all guilty of occasionally overlooking our partner's qualities and neglecting his needs. Sometimes it's just a matter of being busy, but now and then we need to slow down and reinforce our partner's feelings of desirability. As we've said, the world has a way of making all of us feel inadequate. You have the power to convince your man otherwise.

Ask yourself this question: When was the last time you told your partner what a truly wonderful man he is? When was the last time you told him how funny he is or how well he built that bookshelf in the den? When did you last flatter his sexual skills and desirability? If it's been a while, don't panic. This lube job is a quick fix for those men who are running low on sexual compliments. Through a process of flattery, fondling, and fellatio, you'll assure your man that his jewels shine brighter than all the others, and in so doing, you'll reaffirm your love and adoration for him as a partner, both in and out of the bedroom.

Flattery, particularly sexual flattery, is a powerful aphrodisiac. Be honest with yourself. Don't you feel more desirable and more attracted to your partner when he comments on the softness of your skin or the perfect shape of your breasts? Be generous with your praise and heartfelt in your actions. When your partner is in need of maintenance sex, always react with admiration instead of irritation. Rather than acting like his needs are an inconvenience to you, smother him with compliments about his strong libido and tell him how happy you are to have such a hot-blooded man.

Remember that you have the power to build your man up or to tear him down, so choose wisely. It's all in your attitude. If you find your attitude is negative, examine why and correct the problem.

Penis praise is the most direct way to boost your man's sexual ego, and this lube job is the perfect vehicle to deliver those much-needed compliments. This quickie is also a great way to perform maintenance when you're too tired to expend a lot of energy; you get to lie on your back the whole time you play mechanic!

This lube job begins before bedtime. Sprinkle some compliments throughout the day, perhaps admiring your man's broad shoulders or commenting on how sexy he looks when he shaves. When it's time to turn in, lie on your back on the bed and unexpectedly pull your partner down on top of you. Treat him to a long, deep, enticing kiss to catch him off guard and get things started quickly.

Gradually move your kisses down your partner's body, from his mouth to his neck to his chest, either lifting or removing his shirt as you slither downward. Place feathery kisses down the centerline of his body and over his bare stomach until you reach his groin. Reach up to rub his hips and outer and inner thighs before turning your attention to his genitals. Give them a massage while they are underneath his clothing, commenting how good they feel against your hands. Now grab his buttocks, using them as leverage to pull your face up to his groin to kiss his genitals, again while they are still underneath his pants.

When you feel him harden, unzip his pants and push them down just far enough so that you can do your job. Mouth the bulge over the fabric of his underwear, and then push them down out of the way as well. Make a spectacle of the unveiling. Squirm underneath him and tell him how delicious his genitals look. If you can, use a little dirty talk; it's a far greater turn-on for a man to be told his cock is beautiful, than his genitals.

Fondle his penis and testicles for a moment, then grab his buttocks again and pull his groin down toward your face until you can take the head of his penis into your mouth. Suck and tongue just the head. Put your hands on your man's hips and keep them there so you can control how much of his penis goes into your mouth.

Bit by bit, take more of your man's length into your mouth. Pull down on his hips, giving him permission to thrust deeper into your mouth. If he's too eager or goes too deep, gently push up on his hips to have him ease up. By allowing your man to actively penetrate your mouth rather than just passively receive oral sex, you'll give him a nasty feeling of sexual control that he'll love; however, if you don't trust his discipline to obey your hands-on-hips guidance, have him crouch, unmoving, above you while you bring your mouth up to him.

Come on, try just a bite. Some men love the feel of soft nibbles along the length of the shaft and on the head of the penis. If you haven't tried this mouth move before, warn your man in advance and, once you have his okay, treat his penis like the delicacy it is.

Take a break every now and then to praise your partner's man parts. Tell him how sexy he looks crouched above you, how hard and thick he feels in your mouth, and how you can't wait to taste him when he comes.

Pick up the pace by letting your man thrust as deeply as you're comfortable with and at a speed and rhythm you both like. If you're confident he won't lose control and gag you, you can let go of his hips and use one or both hands to squeeze his penis as he pumps into your mouth and nears orgasm.

You can either let him ejaculate into your mouth or, if you prefer, take his penis out of your mouth and stroke it with your hands when you know he's close to climaxing. (You may feel like you're going to choke if you're flat on your back and he comes in your mouth; only you can determine this.) At the very least, lift your head or otherwise shift your position so you aren't lying completely flat on the bed when the moment comes. Your man won't notice some minor last-minute adjusting.

Compliment your man on his superior performance but save a little room for self-flattery, too. You deserve it, for you're a woman who does more than maintain her man in the bedroom, as important as that is. You're also a loving partner who understands the power you have over your man's sexual and personal confidence, and who has decided to use that power to build him—and your relationship—up to towering heights.

Lube Job #8

●

Under the Hood

Women love romantic dinners. We love the soft music, the sweet talk, the cheesecake, and the sparkle in our lover's eyes as he admires us from across the private, candlelit, linen-draped table for two. Men love what comes after dinner. Indeed, there's some truth to the expression "the way to a man's heart is through his stomach," and this tasty lube job puts a new spin on that old saying by chasing a sexy dish with an even sexier dessert that'll have your man licking his lips in satisfaction.

Barb and Gordon are a busy middle-aged couple who own a thriving restaurant in a trendy district of a large city. Their restaurant's enviable location means that they not only have a highly successful business, but also that they cater to a wide and sometimes very unique customer base. It was the exploits of two of their regular customers that demonstrate just how sexy a supper can be.

As Barb relates, this particular couple dined in their restaurant once or twice a month, always late at night and always at a reserved private table in the back of the establishment. They would specifically request that the waiter not disturb them during their meal, and although Barb assumed this was just to ensure a quiet meal, she eventually discovered the real reason. One night, as she stole a quick glance behind the drawn curtain that separated their table from the rest of the restaurant, she was only mildly surprised to see just her male patron at the table. He was sitting back in his chair with the long tablecloth moving below him.

Because the couple always acted discreetly (and left large tips), Barb respected their privacy and let them continue to get their thrills at her restaurant. In fact, she ultimately decided to serve up a little of what they were having at her own table.

"Gord and I spend almost all our time at the restaurant," says Barb. "We usually eat our suppers there after closing and then don't get home until midnight or one o'clock in the morning. By that time I'm too distracted to think about sex. Gord's usually game, but I'm still balancing the till and scheduling employees in my head, so I'm just not into it. He can turn it all off easier than I can."

So, one evening after the restaurant had closed and Gord was sitting alone at a corner table, munching on some cold zucchini sticks and reviewing the new lease agreement, Barb served a dessert that wasn't on the menu. She slipped under the table, and, well, you know the rest.

"I always knew I went into business with the right girl," says Gordon, "but when Barb did that, I knew I married the right girl too. There were many nights we'd get home and I'd want to have sex, but I knew Barb's mind was elsewhere. She handles a lot more of the business side than I do. She does the works, everything from counting eggs to hiring and firing. I'd feel guilty that I was asking for sex, so I wouldn't push it, but then I'd be kind of frustrated that she didn't offer. The night she first went under the table was like something from a movie. I could hardly believe it was happening. It was fantastic."

"I thought I'd feel like an idiot doing it," says Barb, "but I didn't, not at all. It was exciting. Even though we knew the restaurant was all locked up and empty, we could still pretend we were a couple taking that risk in public. Sometimes I'd be giving Gord a blow job under the table just for maintenance purposes, but then I'd get stimulated doing it and we'd end up having intercourse right there on the floor, like a couple of newlyweds."

Barb and Gordon's under-the-table trysts are evidence of a simple fact: one of the easiest and most exciting ways to spice up your sexual routine is to have sex in an unusual place. A change of scenery is sometimes enough to recharge a waning sex drive, but this doesn't mean you have to join the mile-high club or go down on each other in the local movie theater (please don't). For many of us, an unusual place is any place outside the bedroom, and the kitchen is a great place to start.

With a little preparation, even the most utilitarian kitchen table can become a romantic table for two. Throw a nice tablecloth over it to hide any telltale crayon marks, add a few candles and some low classical music to the mix, and serve up a libido-enhancing meal that will satisfy your man's hunger in the best of ways. Why limit maintenance sex to the mattress? That kitchen table of yours holds a lot of erotic potential you can use to pleasure your man.

> **Can't take another bite? Instead of an under-the-table blow job, give your jaw a rest and treat your man to a hand job instead. Put some lube in a bowl and use it as a frisky finger dish to stroke him to climax under the table.**

There's a strong association between food and friskiness that almost every culture recognizes, and you can use this connection to your advantage. Certain foods are believed to have aphrodisiac qualities, though whether or not they actually possess such powers may be irrelevant. The power of suggestion is often enough to get the juices flowing. Better still, some of the most sensual foods are blissfully easy to prepare, which means you can save your creative energy for what you serve under the table rather than expend it on what you put on top of it.

For an easy model menu, serve oysters as appetizers, steak as the main course, and steamed asparagus dressed in butter or olive oil on the side. For dessert, have apricots, strawberries, and/or bananas dipped in warm chocolate or cool whipped cream. Serve wine with supper, and coffee with dessert. Keep the menu simple but sexy. Of course, you'll amend this menu to your tastes, convenience, and cooking ability. If you're a gourmet, the sky's the limit. If, however, your cooking ability is limited to dialing for take-out, no matter. Order anchovies and shrimp on your pizza and call it seafood.

> Money may not grow on trees, but avocados—just picture them—are known as the fruit of the testicle tree and are believed to have aphrodisiac qualities.

As you dine by candlelight (perhaps wearing only lingerie), explain the aphrodisiac qualities of your meal to your partner. He'll be thinking sexy thoughts with each and every bite. Tell him that seafood, including the oysters he's eating, is believed to increase a man's libido because Aphrodite, the goddess of love, was born of the sea. When he bites into that juicy steak, tell him how the protein in steak also increases a man's sexual energy. Then hold up a piece of that oh-so-phallic asparagus, and lick the butter off the tip as you throw him a flirtatious wink. Take a sip of wine, and tell him how alcohol is the most common aphrodisiac. It lowers inhibitions and sets desires free. Tell him how the ancients used to have sexual orgies, bacchanals, where they'd drink and have sex with whoever they wanted, all thanks to the god of wine, Bacchus.

As you're delighting in the tastes and smells of your sex supper, flirt often and openly with your partner. Play footsies under the table and lean over to let him sneak a peek at the curves of your breasts. Keep the dinner conversation focused on sexual aphrodisiacs to increase his arousal. It's a fun topic, so you shouldn't have much difficulty holding his attention. You can talk about the millions of dollars that are spent every year as people search for that magic love potion in everything from creams to perfumes to power drinks.

> Abstinence can be an effective aphrodisiac. Every now and then, neglect your maintenance duties for an extra night to let your man's desire for you really build. Just don't shirk your responsibilities too often, or you'll go from arousing to aggravating. And make sure your partner knows your hands-off approach is foreplay, not forgetfulness.

When it's time for dessert, dip your fruit in chocolate or whipped cream and teasingly lick it off as your partner watches. If you're having bananas, dip a whole one in cream and suck it off. He'll get the idea. To press the point, you can dip his fingers in cream and suck them clean as well. Twirl your tongue around the palm of his hand to exploit this very erogenous area. Ask your partner to empty his coffee cup, since caffeine is a stimulant. Tell him that you want him wide awake for what comes next.

If you're still in the mood for sweets, take the whipping cream and/or chocolate with you, and, with a devilish smile, disappear under the table. Run your hands up your partner's legs, over his thighs, to his groin. Unfasten his pants and expose his genitals, then place soft kisses around his groin area, from his thighs and hips to his penis and testicles, to arouse him.

"Food can give a person so many enjoyable feelings," says Barb, "and I learned to use it under the table, too. Sometimes I'd put a warm dessert sauce on Gord's penis and lick it off, then I'd put something cool on it, like whipping cream, just to give him different feelings down there. It's an erotic thing to do."

If you wish, you can follow Barb's lead and use the whipping cream and/or chocolate to complement oral sex. Just remember that the skin on a man's penis is extremely sensitive, so be careful and don't apply anything that is too warm or too cool. Experiment by going slowly at first and only proceeding if your partner likes what's going on under the hood. Spread the sweets of your choice over his penis and take your time licking them off. Why rush a good meal?

> **If you don't want to use food on your partner's privates, purchase a selection of flavored lubricants and put them on the table as if they were on the menu. Let him choose the flavors you get to sample.**

When this down-below dessert is finished, you can bring the meal to a delicious end by proceeding to full-blown fellatio. Receiving oral sex in this unusual and intensely erotic way will be a real thrill for your man, so let him sit back and lose himself in the sensations. Let him ejaculate in your mouth to make this the finest dining experience he's ever had, start to finish.

"It's a total fantasy, there's nothing like it," says Gordon. "Having all those feelings going on down there but not being able to see them just takes your breath away. I can't tell you how good it feels. I sit back in the chair, spread my legs, and I'm in heaven. It's fairly dirty, too, and I can't say that doesn't turn me on. My mind wanders, and I sometimes pretend we're out in public and she's gone down on me. That makes the whole experience even more unbelievable. She's done it lots of times, but every time is like the first. I can't get enough of it, and I think those are the strongest orgasms I have."

But what about the hardworking chef, you ask. Where's the thanks for making such a mouthwatering meal? According to Barb, the gratitude you'll receive goes well beyond the standard twenty-percent gratuity.

"Real gratitude isn't a few dollars left behind by a stranger," she says. "Real gratitude is the way your husband looks at you and hugs you when you do something like this for him. In my opinion, maintenance sex isn't a thankless job, not if you have a good man. And if you're fortunate enough to have a good man, like I do, you get back way more than you put into it."

Lube Job #9

●

Grab a Gear—Part II: The Detour

Is sexual boredom inevitable in a long-term relationship? Does familiarity, as the saying goes, breed contempt?

"It was the socks that did it," says Mirriam. "Right there, in the middle of the kitchen floor. He was standing sockless by the stove, slurping the last of the white wine sauce right from the pot."

Mirriam and Nicholas had been living together for ten years, and over the past decade things had become a bit . . . um . . . relaxed.

"I made a romantic 'ten years together' dinner, and we ate by candlelight," explains Mirriam. "I wanted to take the evening slow, but Nick knocked back his food like he was late for a flight. After the feeding frenzy I excused myself to slip into something more comfortable, and when I came back in a garter, he was standing barefoot beside the stove, holding the pot to his lips, guzzling my gourmet sauce like a cold beer. The socks were there, lying in a heap in the middle of the floor, almost symbolic."

Her partner's faux pas notwithstanding, Mirriam was determined to stay in a sexy mood. She asked Nick what movies he had rented for their special anniversary evening. "Two kung fu movies and a horror flick," recalls Mirriam. "I felt like I was trapped in a bad sitcom. The only thing missing was the fake laugh track. Nick finally put down the pot and noticed me standing there wearing this garter thing. I suddenly felt ridiculous, like I was trying to be twenty years younger than I was, but he whistled like a construction worker and swept me off my feet. He was all over me, but as hard as I tried, I just couldn't get into it. Thank goodness for lube."

The next day, Mirriam was relating her anniversary antics to her female co-workers, sharing and laughing about the flames-to-fizzle progression that seemed to characterize long-term relationships.

"It was unanimous," Mirriam says, "all my colleagues felt the same way: very much in love, totally devoted to their partners, but losing those sparks of sexual attraction. Most of us had partners or husbands who were still sexually attracted to us, but we had lost the motivation to fulfill their needs. I used to get butterflies when Nick would touch me unexpectedly, but that wasn't happening as much. You do your best to get the spark back, whether it's buying sexy teddies or going away for a weekend, but it's hard when your reality is socks in the middle of the floor. You're just so familiar with him—and his underwear—that it's hard to see him as the stud you first fell for. Now he's your life partner and you love him, but you miss those butterflies."

For some women, this is the time in their long-term relationship when maintenance sex becomes particularly laborious, not necessarily because they don't want to do it but because they simply don't have the sexual motivation they once did. Plainly said, they aren't as turned on by their partner as they used to be. This time can be fraught with other dangers as well, from emotional and physical disconnection to relationship ambivalence and infidelity.

> **GONE BUT NOT FORGOTTEN**
> The hormone-charged honeymoon phase can last from weeks to years, but don't lament its loss when it's gone. Instead, keep it alive by fondly remembering the early feelings, excitement, and experiences you and your partner shared during this sweet and special time in your relationship.

"I knew my relationship was strong," says Mirriam. "I knew exactly what was happening. Those sex hormones, the adrenaline rush of a new lover were gone, and we were settling into each other."

But "settling into each other" isn't necessarily a bad thing. As a relationship progresses, the erotic tingles of newness may lessen, but other more valuable and enduring qualities, such as security, comfort, and deep love, thrive. If a couple is aware of what is happening in their relationship and why it is happening, they can take steps to ensure that their sex life remains healthy and happy and that those tingles don't disappear. Sadly, however, not everyone is so astute.

"Alicia was a young wife in our office who was married for just a year," says Mirriam. "It seemed soon, but she was always complaining about losing sexual interest in her husband. Nobody was surprised when she began to flirt with a male co-worker."

According to Mirriam, the new wife's flirtation started innocently enough, with a warm smile, a wink, or a sassy text message. But just as the older women in the office predicted, the play grew more serious until the couple was stepping out for long lunches together, exchanging lingering looks across the room, and finding any excuse to visit each other's office—behind closed doors, of course.

"We all knew exactly what was happening," says Mirriam, "and we knew why. We had all felt the sizzle fade a bit in our relationships, but we were smart enough to know it was natural. We warned Alicia that she was playing a dangerous game, but she just waved us off. We told her the sizzle will fade no matter who you're with and that you're wiser to keep it going instead of starting it up somewhere else. She said she was just looking for a little excitement and a way to pass the time at work. She said her sex life was better with her husband because this guy at work gave her a thrill. But just like we warned, it turned into an affair. The whole thing got messy and very sad."

Yet the young co-worker's misery became Mirriam's motivation.

"Watching Alicia's experience made me appreciate my relationship all the more," says Mirriam. "I was so proud

> Rather than flirting with that suave new co-worker, reserve your efforts for your man. Flirting doesn't have to go the way of the dodo once the honeymoon's over. Touch your man often, plant unexpected kisses on the back of his neck, tell him you love him, and lift your skirt to give him a sassy peek. Keep playfulness in your long-term relationship, and let him know he still turns you on, even after all these years. What a stud he must be!

of Nick and me for reaching our tenth anniversary and still being in love, socks on the floor and all. I had renewed motivation. I wanted to get those butterflies back and to feel excited by him. He wasn't asking for sex as much as he used to, although I knew he still wanted it. He was sensing my indifference, and that must have been hurting him. He deserved better, and I wanted to give him better."

But how to get those butterflies back? For Mirriam, it was a casual trip to the mall that showed her the way. Valentine's Day was a few weeks away, and the shops were advertising their "For Him" wares in abundance. As she strolled down the aisles of her favorite department store, something caught her eye or, rather, her nose.

"I went down the fragrance aisle, and I was enveloped by the scent of men's cologne," says Mirriam. "It smelled so good, so sexy. I put some on my wrist, took a good whiff, and within moments I was becoming aroused thinking about it on Nick. I've always been turned on by a man wearing cologne, but I realized it had been years since Nick had worn any. He didn't even own a bottle anymore."

Mirriam bought the cologne, but she didn't stop there. She also bought Nicholas a closet full of new clothes, including a trendy hoody, a good suit, stylish jeans, and a number of shirts she knew he'd look and feel handsome in.

"Nick's not the kind of guy to shop for himself," Mirriam says, "but like any of us, he likes to look good. He loved the clothes and was very appreciative that I'd taken the time to shop just for him. This was just icing on the cake, because when he was all decked out in his new clothes, smelling so sexy, I was incredibly attracted to him. I remembered how gorgeous he was and how sexy I found him. Just seeing him in new clothes and smelling him in a new scent was enough to kick-start my libido. For me, it really was that easy."

As an extra bonus, Nicholas's makeover had an unexpected effect on their relationship. Feeling good about himself and appreciative of his woman, Nicholas too began to feel a resurgence of romantic attraction to his long-time partner. Date nights became weekly events. Once, he even passed right by a newly released kung fu movie to pick a romantic comedy off the shelf.

But what about the socks?

"They're still on the floor," admits Mirriam, "and with any luck, they'll be there for many years to come."

While familiarity may not always breed contempt, it can lead to a loss of sexual interest in one's partner, particularly in long-term relationships. Most women experience ups and downs in their sexual attraction to their longtime partner, but for many women in otherwise healthy relationships, the "downs" can be lifted with just a little effort. For Mirriam, it was as simple as seeing (and smelling) her partner in a new way. His wardrobe makeover was enough to remind her how handsome and sexy he was and to bring back the tingles.

> To keep your relationship dynamic, bring new beginnings into it. For example, start a new health regime together, buy dirt bikes and take up the fun sport, sign up for a cooking or wine-tasting class, or learn a second language together.

If you're in love with your partner yet sometimes feel ambivalent about sex, consider trying the Mirriam Makeover yourself. Like its namesake, you may find that this simple strategy is enough to rekindle your attraction to your man. That in turn may give you the sexual motivation you need to kick-start your love life and satisfy all your partner's sexual needs. But don't stop with new clothes or different cologne. Your approach to maintenance sex may need a wardrobe change, too.

Too often maintenance sex is performed without any variety: in bed, late at night, either flat on our backs or with tired hands tugging away. No wonder women dread it, and men don't get any satisfaction beyond basic relief. Instead, save the warm comfort of your bed for long lovemaking sessions and think outside the bedroom box when it comes to maintenance. Give your relationship a maintenance sex makeover. How, you ask? Hit the road.

This lube job exploits the excitement of sex in the car, but unlike Part I, Part II ups the ante by adding oral sex to the jackpot. Car sex is great for maintenance since it's fast, spontaneous, raunchy, and lots of fun. Receiving a blow job in the driver's seat is something that every man with a driver's license has fantasized about, so it's an ideal way to turbocharge your maintenance sex routine. You may even find that performing maintenance sex in different ways and places will thrill you as much as your partner does.

If you have a long road trip coming up, save this lube job for the jaunt. Otherwise, proposition your partner for a late-night drive. Choose a night when you know he'll be looking for love. Sometimes the simplest things in life are the sweetest: an unplanned evening drive with your man can be more romantic than an elaborate night out. It gives you the opportunity to speak privately, without interruption, and the physical closeness can be very special. It's disturbing just how little time we actually spend shoulder to shoulder with our true loves. As you're driving along, reach down to caress your partner's thigh, gradually moving your fingers toward his groin. Lean close to him and rub your palm over his bulge until he begins to harden.

Remember, if your man is becoming aroused he's also getting distracted. Find a safe, secluded spot to park and pull over before you grab his gear. Ask him to push his seat back as you unfasten his pants and push down his underwear. Focus on his arousal and the excitement of what you're doing. The more you enjoy the experience, the more turned-on your partner will be. The novelty and dirtiness of what you're doing, combined with the muffled sounds in the car and the potential for exposure, should have your hearts pounding with pleasure.

Caress your man's groin with your fingertips and then lean over into his lap. Breathe hotly onto the head of his penis, then trace around it with the tip of your tongue. Lick down his shaft toward the base of his penis. Don't use your hands; just stimulate him with your tongue and lips by licking and kissing along his length. Making sure that your lips are covering your teeth, take the head of his penis in your mouth and suck on it before swallowing as much of his shaft as you can. Suck as you move your lips back up his length, but don't pull your mouth off as you reach the top. Instead, keep just the head of his penis in your mouth and spend some time sucking and licking it before again stroking downward.

Now for the detour. Sit back up in your seat and tell your partner to drive to a second location. Or, if his mind is no longer focused on the road, hop into the driver's seat yourself and chauffeur him to the next destination. It doesn't matter where—whether it's a specific address or another secluded destination—but let him know that when he gets there you'll be ready to finish what you've started. The detour will delay his gratification and increase the strength of his orgasm. It'll also give you time to anticipate going back down on him.

Let the sexual tension mount as you drive to the next locale. You can make the trip a challenge by choosing a difficult address to find, but if you're more merciful, select somewhere quick and easy. As always, use common sense and discretion when selecting a spot for car sex. It's hard to feel sexy if you don't feel safe. Moreover, the thrill of being watched should always remain a fantasy. The reality would be embarrassing at best and criminal at worst. Secure, unpopulated areas are your best bet.

If you think an unpopulated area diminishes excitement, think again. Total privacy gives you the freedom to open the door, quite literally, to added fun. When you're parked in a quiet spot where you're confident you won't be busted, jump out of the car and go to the driver's side door. Open the door and ask your man to sit sideways in his seat so that his feet are planted on the ground, and then kneel down between his legs to pleasure him in this exposed position. You'll both love the erotic sense of exhibitionism.

This road trip can take as many detours as you wish to prolong the pleasure, but don't overdo it. Making your man wait too long for release can go from foreplay to frustration before you even realize it. When you're ready to end the journey, find the sucking and stroking rhythm that will build your partner's orgasm, add your hands to the mix for extra friction and pressure, and don't let up until he comes.

See? Wasn't that more fun than that old why-is-this-taking-so-long duty tug at bedtime? You had some fresh air, a nice drive, pleasant conversation, gave a great blow job, and maybe even had some drive-thru onion rings on the ride home. Best of all, you showed your man that you don't regard fulfilling his sexual needs as a dreaded chore, but rather as an opportunity to have fun, satisfy him, and strengthen your loving relationship. So take a good long look in the mirror and see if your relationship is in need of a maintenance sex makeover.

A makeover is a mighty thing. To recharge your bedroom's sex appeal, do a romantic room makeover. Choose colors, lighting, furniture, bedding, and fabrics that create an aura of sensuality, intimacy, and passion. After all, your bedroom is your biggest erogenous zone.

Lube Job #10

●

The Engine Soak

When we were writing the proposal for this book, we spent a lot of time thinking about which issues negatively affect long-term relationships, love lives, and maintenance sex. In the process, we visited a few online message boards where women meet to discuss common relationship problems (everything from video-game-addicted boyfriends to unfaithful husbands). One topic really had us talking, not because it complemented our book's focus, but because it challenged it. When we think of disparate sex drives, we usually assume the man wants more and the woman wants less; however, we were surprised to find a number of discussions where women were lamenting their male partner's lack of libido.

It seemed that the majority of the women discussing this topic took their mate's drop in desire personally. They feared that their partner was not attracted to them anymore; that they had gained weight, become too boring or familiar, or weren't good lovers. When Don asked me if I too would take the *occasional* sexual rejection personally, I had to say yes, despite his wholehearted assurances that any number of things could temporarily distract him from sex. He said I was being paranoid. I told him I was being normal. So, what was it: normal or paranoid?

As usual, I began to make some calls. After all, a consensus among like-minded girlfriends holds more weight than a month-long, jury-deliberated, DNA-backed not guilty verdict. As Don sighed and shook his head, I phoned every woman I knew: all ages, married, single, divorced, kids, no kids, pets, no pets, piercings, no piercings. You get the picture. I asked each woman the simple question "If your partner sexually rejected you tonight, would you take it personally?"

The results of my inherently flawed, completely informal, and embarrassingly unreliable supper-hour telephone survey? Fifteen women said yes, they'd take it personally. A confident six—the sexually sage, perhaps—said no, not necessarily, since other factors may be to blame. One hang-up. I guess that translates to my being seventy-one percent normal, twenty-nine percent paranoid. Actually, I think that's pretty damn accurate.

Since I don't believe in coincidence, I shouldn't have been surprised when a short time later my musings were put to the test. We had just sold the book, and I was busy scribbling a first draft. Don was working a grueling overtime stretch of twenty-one fourteen-hour days in a row: gone at six A.M., back at eight or nine P.M. Our son came down with a nasty stomach bug from his preschool; my mother needed surgery; and one of Don's dearest friends passed away. It all happened within a short period of time, and for the first time since we brought our son home from the hospital four years earlier, our sex life began to fade into the background. That's right, smack in the middle of writing a sex guide.

But there was one difference between the dry spell four years ago and this sudden drought. This time it was Don who was too distracted to think dirty. Ouch. I was right; I took it one-hundred-percent personally, despite his assertions that he was just feeling overworked, exhausted, stressed out, anxious, and a little depressed. It would pass, he told me. It was nothing to do with me; he just couldn't flip the work switch in his head to off. By next week, he said, we'd be back to normal and I'd be beating him away with a stick.

> **Give the man some elbow room. If he comes home stressed or in a foul mood, give him space before you swarm in with questions or words of support. Our girlfriends might want to share and "talk about it" right away, but our men often want some alone time to ruminate before discussion period begins. Tell him you'll be there to listen when he's ready to talk, then back off. You'll have his appreciation and his confidence.**

I knew he was right. It was an uncharacteristically stressful time, and we both knew it would soon pass and our sex life would return to normal. That didn't mean I couldn't try to help the process along, though. I thought about the many times I had felt overwhelmed, whether because of school, work, or the baby, when Don had come to my rescue by sharing my stress. Whenever I was extremely distracted, he would do the simplest but *sexiest* thing: he would run a hot bath and sit in the tub with me while I soaked my cares away. (This has to be one of the top five reasons I love this man!)

Even though he's a devout shower man, I decided to give Don a dose of his own tub therapy to help him through this stressful but sexless time. Just before we were ready to turn in for the night, I slipped into the bathroom and ran a hot bath. I dimmed the lights and set his favorite car magazine by the side of the tub. When he asked if I was having a bath, I said yes and asked him to join me; however, I said I wanted just to relax and wind down, not do anything sexual.

We lay in the bath for some time, while Don read his magazine to me and I feigned interest in the many advantages of air-cooled Volkswagen engines. I didn't want him to think about work, loss, and especially not sex. I wanted him to relax in a completely undemanding and nonsexual way. Had he felt any pressure to perform sexually, I knew my attempts to calm him would have had the opposite effect. As I expected, his mood improved. He began to breath easier, laugh easier, and the world beyond the closed bathroom door seemed to disappear.

Taking a risk, I reached for some papers on the sink and casually handed them to him. "This is a rough draft of an erotic story I'm working on for the book," I told him. "Do you want to take a peek? It can wait if you're not in

> ✺ **Take care of yourself. Do your best to maintain a healthy body weight and lifestyle, and encourage your man to do the same. Health greatly affects an individual's level of sexual desire, which in turn can affect the quality of a couple's sex life.**

the mood." As I lay back on his body, he began to read it. What happened from there stays behind closed doors.

The truth is, men are under a lot of pressure to perform like sexual machines. It's a bit of a double standard. If a woman goes through an occasional period of being uninterested in sex, it's no big deal. In fact, it's considered completely normal and expected. But if a man is uninterested, well, let the guessing games begin: Is he impotent? Cheating? Do I turn him off? Is he looking at too much porn? Is he getting old? What's the problem, dammit? What's wrong with you? What's wrong with *me*?

If your man is going through a period where he seems less interested in sex, try not to jump to self-conscious conclusions. Instead, step back and take a look at the big picture. What's going on at work? Has he just had an argument with his brother? Is he worried about your finances or his health? If so, the best thing to do might be nothing at all. Good communication is essential to a strong relationship, but sometimes the best communication is silence. If you're anything like me, that's an excruciating order, but the last thing you want to do is compound your man's stress by adding sexual pressure to his list of problems.

Instead, focus on relaxing your man's mind and body. If sex follows, great; if it doesn't, it will soon enough. Just don't let on that it's your goal. Think about maintenance sex in a larger sense. While it's usually about satisfying his sexual abundance, it can also be about watering his sexual droughts, sheltering him from feelings of inadequacy, and managing his stress. Like exhaustion and insecurity, stress is a deterrent to sexual arousal. When your man's mind is preoccupied with work or worries, sex is the last thing he has on the brain. That's why you have to do the thinking.

You know how to best alleviate your man's stress. Does he like golf? Encourage him to spend a day on the green with a buddy. Does he like movies? Pick up tickets for the latest guy flick and cuddle in the theater and during the car ride home, but let him initiate anything more intimate. Or, send him down to the basement to hide out and enjoy a James Bond marathon on his own. You can even try a soak in the tub, whether solo or partnered. If a hard-core shower man like Don can gear down in the water, maybe your man can, too. Just don't girl-out on him: skip the bubble bath and don't even try to put sliced cucumber on his eyelids.

> **Curb the complaining.** If he's irritated and says the boss is nagging him, make sure he doesn't mean you. Suppress that female nag gene (unless it's really warranted) and bite your tongue when he yet again ignores that dripping tap in the bathroom.

Sharing a bath is a delightful way to spend some soothing yet sensual downtime with your partner in the serenity of your own bathroom, and its advantages are many. It's an effective stress buster that'll get you through those unexpected life crises, but it's also an equally effective way to keep stress at bay on a regular basis by preventing those everyday worries and irritations from flaring out of control. Like the practice of sensual massage (see chapter 19) sharing a bath can also sustain your emotional and physical connection as a couple and provide you with an opportunity to perform some exquisitely erotic maintenance sex on your man.

To get the most out of this steamy lube job, you should first make your bathroom a suitable venue for the event. This doesn't mean installing heated imported Italian tile floors or elaborate artificial rock waterfalls. Even the most unadorned bathroom can be transformed by switching off the harsh hundred-watters and lighting some scented candles. A few tea lights placed at various spots in your bathroom will create a comforting, alluring ambience that is as romantic as it is relaxing. Bath kits come complete with everything from candles to milk soaks and can be convenient one-stop shopping.

Also, invest in a thick, fluffy bath mat. It'll feel luxurious under your and your partner's bare feet. Countertop or wall-mounted water fountains are also widely available and inexpensive and, when lit by candlelight, can make your powder room a private heaven. If you don't have a jet tub, there are low-cost portable jet units that can be mounted to your bathtub to add the luxury of pulsing water to the experience.

If you'd like, set two glasses of wine or cups of herbal tea by the tub. You can even have ready chocolate-dipped strawberries or another sweet, sexy favorite. A stack of your man's favorite magazines should also be close by, and it wouldn't hurt to have this book within arm's reach, too; the erotica from chapter 16 can heat up the water if it starts to cool off. Run a hot bath (place a towel under the door to retain the room's humidity) and slip into the sea with your man.

Don't rush the festivities. Lie back on your man while he soaks, relaxes, reads, unwinds. Talk about the things that interest him. In all likelihood, the mood may naturally turn from sensual to sexual, whether he reads the erotica or not; the warmth of the water and the closeness of his woman's naked body may be more than enough to stir his desire.

> **If your partner's drop in sexual desire becomes worrisome, book him an appointment with his physician and, if necessary, drive him to the clinic yourself. The causes and treatments of sexual problems are many, so leave the diagnosing to the pros.**

When you sense your man is getting aroused, move your body against his and let your hands slip under the water to caress him. If he seems to want more, ask him to sit up on the edge of the bathtub and open his legs. Kneel in the tub, between your man's spread knees (you can have him stand up in the tub if that's easier) and wash his genitals. Put your hands on his thighs or hips and hold on to him as you begin to kiss his groin area, particularly his inner thighs, perineum, and scrotum. Nuzzle your face in his pubic hair, brushing his penis with your nose, before placing wet licks along the sensitive underside of his penis, right up to the frenulum.

Take the head of his penis in your mouth and swirl your tongue around it. Using the warm water and your own saliva as lubrication, stroke his penis with your mouth. Hold the base of his penis with one hand and continue to stroke the shaft with your mouth while you caress his testicles and perineum with your other hand, even inching back to stimulate his anus. Drag your fingers down the sides of his waist, brush your hand across his lower belly (the small area between his penis and just below his belly button), then reach around to caress his bum. These are very sensitive spots, and if you touch them with feathery finger strokes you'll increase his arousal.

When you're ready to release his stress in a big way, use a hand-and-mouth combination to stroke and suck him to relief. As his orgasm builds, apply steady pressure to either his anus, if he likes that, or to his perineum. Don't let up on your stroking, sucking, or pressure until well after he's finished coming. You don't want to lower his speed until he's reached his destination.

A bath time blow job is a very sensual form of stress-busting maintenance sex. It's also a good way for women who do not usually perform oral sex to spoil their man. Because you're in the water, you can clean your partner's genitals to your satisfaction. You can also spit his ejaculate into a nearby washcloth or even into the water, and then clean your own mouth immediately afterward. As long as you do this with respect and discretion, he shouldn't mind too much, especially if his blow jobs are few and far between. With all its health benefits and pleasure possibilities, you may find this watery lube job has you and your man skinny-dipping on a regular basis.

Instead of a girly bubble bath or lavender bath oil, try a man-friendly, stress-busting bath soak of Epsom salts. It'll improve his circulation; ease his aches, pains, and worries; and reduce any inflammation or muscle cramping he might have. Two cups in a standard-sized bathtub should be enough to relax both body and mind.

Part Three

Accessories

Lube Job #11

◉

The Roadside Check

Cruise control is a handy thing on a long road trip. Push in that little button, and your car glides effortlessly down the highway. All you have to do is keep one hand on the steering wheel and watch the road. Since we're responsible car owners, we know that the tires have good air pressure, the tank has enough fuel, and the brakes are in good working order. Through regular maintenance, we've ensured that our car is mechanically sound. If a deer suddenly darts across the highway, we're confident we can tap the brakes to slow down and that cruise control will turn off, thereby returning control to us.

Unfortunately, we sometimes use cruise control in our intimate relationships and often far less responsibly than we do on the road. Things are going well enough, so we push in that little button and let our partnership roll along on its own momentum. And while this is safe enough in the car, it's an accident waiting to happen in a relationship.

When was the last time you pulled your relationship over to the side of the road to ensure it is completely sound?

This lube job gives you the opportunity to do just that: to pull over, lift the hood, and check that everything is working. After all, your man may be in need of maintenance without your even knowing it.

Some of the couples' stories featured in this book are based on material we obtained through a questionnaire. The questionnaire was designed for couples in marriages or long-term relationships, and was in three parts: part I was for partners to fill out together; part II was for the woman; and part III was for the man. The questions dealt with common relationship issues, many of which focused on the role of maintenance sex in the relationship, such as the frequency of, the attitude towards, etc. The answers we received were extremely helpful in writing this book, but the questionnaire had an unintended but positive side effect: it encouraged couples to openly discuss how maintenance sex factored into their relationship.

Both female and male respondents expressed gratitude for having been given a *reason* to stop and examine their sex life in a direct way. They also said that the questionnaire gave them a reason and the means to examine their relationship in general. By answering honestly and then sharing their responses, they gained both insight into and sympathy for each other's feelings, stressors, and behaviors. Some couples even said the questionnaire was a bonding exercise. As they worked through the questions, they felt a sense of emotional and sexual solidarity that they hadn't felt in a long while.

Often, our intentions are noble, but our actions aren't equal to the task. Most of us in committed relationships want our partner to be happy, but life has a way of pulling us in so many directions that we don't ever stop to give our partner our undivided attention or to ask whether he's truly satisfied with things the way they are. Are there areas that need work? It's simple maintenance, but when we're flying along on cruise control, it never seems to get done.

Well, it's time to take your relationship off cruise control, pull over, and perform a thorough roadside check. Below, we've included a selection of questions based on those in our original questionnaire. Although some of the questions have been modified and we've obviously omitted those regarding demographics and personal history, we've retained the three-part format of the questionnaire. Not all of the questions may be relevant to all readers, so focus on the ones that apply to your circumstances.

Tonight, instead of surfing the channels on TV, open the channels of communication with your partner by sitting on the bed and completing this sex questionnaire together with honesty, with no holds barred, and with no fear of repercussions.

If you give your man the opportunity to express any dissatisfaction he has with your sex life—and if you do so with a kind heart and loving spirit—you'll be able to see which parts need work and then to fix any damage long before it's irreparable. This questionnaire will also give you the chance to express your feelings to your partner in a nonthreatening way. Of course, it's up to you whether you want to complete parts II and III in each other's company.

It doesn't matter, as long as you give each other permission to be brutally honest in your answers and you agree to share them without prejudice or punishment.

Here are the questions:

PART I

For Couples

1. Small children and/or busy schedules can interfere with a couple's sex life. How do you work in time for sex in light of children and/or busy schedules? Have you made any unusual efforts to ensure you have time for sex?

2. All long-term couples experience ups and downs in their sex lives. What do you do to get the spark back?

3. How many times a week, on average, do you engage in:

    (a) sexual intercourse
    (b) oral sex
    (c) hand jobs
    (d) mutual masturbation

4. Who usually initiates sex?

5. What is the average length of time you spend having sex, including foreplay?

6. What time of the day or night do you usually engage in sexual activity? What is your usual presex routine?

7. What form does foreplay usually take (e.g., erotic massage, kissing, showering together)?

8. What are the most significant issues that, now or in the past, have negatively affected your relationship (e.g., money worries, job stress, an ex-spouse)? Can you detail any specific incidents?

9. What are the most significant issues that, now or in the past, have negatively affected your sex life (e.g., birth of a child, infidelity, poor health, an argument)? Can you detail any specific incidents?

10. How did you resolve the above issue(s) to get your sex life back on track?

11. Other than the bedroom, where are you most likely to have sex? Can you relay a favorite experience that took place outside the bedroom?

PART II

For Her Only

12. Do you ever feel overwhelmed by your daily demands, including work and/or children? Specifically, what overwhelms you?

13. Do you feel the daily grind negatively impacts your sex life? If so, are there things your partner could do to increase your sexual desire? (Yes, that can include housework!)

14. Who is more in control of whether and when you engage in sex, you or your partner?

15. What are some of the main obstacles to sex in your relationship (e.g., relationship problems, differences in level of sexual desire, religious issues)?

16. In terms of frequency, how much sex would satisfy you (e.g., three times a week, once every two weeks, never)?

17. Do you ever perform duty or maintenance sex just to please your partner? If you do, how does it make you feel (e.g., used, loving, indifferent)? If you do not, what are your reasons for not performing maintenance sex?

18. On average, how many times per week do you perform maintenance sex? What does maintenance sex usually involve (e.g., fellatio, intercourse, hand jobs)?

19. Do you ever feel your partner wants sex too often? How does this make you feel (e.g., irritated, flattered)?

20. What is your attitude toward maintenance sex in general? Would you encourage or discourage other women to perform it? Why or why not?

21. Do you ever refuse your partner when you know he wants to have sex? How often and what is his usual reaction?

22. Do you ever feel guilty for not having sex with your partner when he wants to? Why or why not?

23. Overall, how do you feel about your sex life (e.g., satisfied, dissatisfied)? Why?

24. Have you and your partner ever fought about sex? If so, what specifically did you fight about (e.g., frequency, trying something new)?

25. Sexually speaking, what most displeases you about your partner (e.g., he initiates sex too often, doesn't spend enough time in foreplay)?

26. The task of spicing things up in the bedroom often falls to the woman in a relationship. Do you agree with this statement, and how does it make you feel?

27. Have you ever tried to spice things up in the bedroom? If so, how (e.g., sex books, adult films, new lingerie, sex toys)? What was the result?

28. Do you ever worry about your partner either being attracted to another woman or being unfaithful?

29. Do you ever feel that you are not doing enough to keep your partner sexually satisfied? How does that make you feel (e.g., resentful, worried, indifferent)?

30. Does your partner view pornography? If so, what kind (e.g., Internet, magazines, adult films)? How do you feel about this?

(PART III)

For Him Only

31. Do you ever feel overwhelmed by your daily demands, such as work and/or children? What overwhelms you? How is your libido affected?

32. How does your partner's attitude affect your sexual attraction to her?

33. Do you ever feel that your sex life is controlled by your partner? In what way (e.g., her mood swings, level of sexual desire, fatigue, distraction, etc.)?

34. Do you feel more loved when your partner expresses her appreciation for all that you do? Do you ever wish she would express her appreciation more?

35. In terms of frequency, how much sex would satisfy you (e.g., every day, three times a week, once a month)?

36. Do you ever wish your partner would engage in sex more often? If so, do you ever masturbate in lieu of sex: (a) never, (b) rarely, or (c) regularly?

37. Are you aware when you partner is engaging in so-called maintenance sex? What tips you off?

38. What is your attitude toward maintenance sex? Do you think a woman should regularly practice it to keep her man satisfied? Why or why not?

39. How often do you think about sex (e.g., every day, several times a day)?

40. What is your favorite sexual position or activity?

41. Do you wish your partner would initiate sex more often? How would it make you feel if she did?

42. When you're feeling stress, do you want more or less sex? Why?

43. Does your partner ever refuse you when you want sex? If so, how does this make you feel (e.g., angry, resentful, hurt, rejected)?

44. Have you and your partner ever fought about sex? If so, what specifically did you fight about (e.g., frequency, trying something new)?

45. Do you ever feel sexually frustrated or unfulfilled? If so, how does that affect your mood or emotions (e.g., feel more irritable or stressed, less loved)?

46. Sexually speaking, are there things you want to try but are hesitant to suggest? If so, what are they (e.g., a new position, sex toys, adult films)?

47. In your opinion, how important is a good sex life to a lasting relationship? Do you feel emotionally closer to your partner when your sex life is satisfying?

48. What things does your partner do that turn you on (e.g., fellatio, wear sexy lingerie, flatter you)?

49. **What things does your partner do that turn you off (e.g., talk about the kids, lack sexual enthusiasm, nag)?**

50. **How do you think your sex life could be improved (e.g., more adventurous, less predictable, more frequency)?**

Once you've completed the questionnaire, get set to share your answers for Parts II and III. The insight you gain by doing so will make you more sensitive and sympathic to the nonsexual stresses (such as work, kids, and finances) that indirectly affect each other's sexuality. Your man may be surprised to learn how much more sexual energy you'd have in the bedroom if he would help clean up in the kitchen. And you may be surprised to learn how much his stress level at work is reduced when he is sexually satisfied at home. The more you discuss your answers, the more you will understand each other's perspective, and the more you can negotiate changes in your sex life that will please both of you.

Now that you and your partner have entered into this new and exciting era of sexual openness, you can safely proceed to the next phase of this lube job, that is, the sex itself. After you've finished discussing what may be some heavy answers, you can lighten things up by reaching under the bed and pulling out your own personalized toolbox. What's inside? Why, sex tools, of course. There's no point identifying those body parts that need work if you aren't going to repair them.

Tell your partner that all this talk about maintenance sex has put you in the servicing mood. Open your sex toolbox with him and explore the lusty contents. Use a real toolbox. It's a fun idea and the perfect shape for stowing away sex toys. Your toolbox can contain anything you'd like, from a simple feather to high-tech sex toys. Since other lube jobs in this book feature a penis sleeve, a straight vibrator, blindfold and restraints, a remote-controlled bullet vibrator, as well as different types of personal lubricants, massage oils, and bath kits, you may want to include these items.

Other items to consider are: a penis ring, nipple clamps, a dildo, novelty condoms, sweet treats, and adult videos and skin magazines. Slightly more adventurous toys include penis pumps and a host of anal toys from butt plugs to anal beads. These will be discussed in turn, below.

> **Water-based lubricants are recommended for most sex toys since their ingredients won't damage latex or silicone. They're also the most pleasant and wash off easily with soap and water. And even though the better brands are long lasting, if they do dry out, they can be reconstituted with water.**

A penis or cock ring is an essential for any sex toolbox. This common male toy can be as simple as a rubber circle or as elaborate as a softly flexible vibrating ring with extensions to tease a woman's clitoris during intercourse. You can buy adjustable or nonadjustable, and even disposables that vibrate. Regardless of the options, the standard model is a ring that fits snugly around the base of the penis, or under the scrotum if your man prefers. The ring helps a man maintain his erection by stopping blood flow out of an erect penis. It also adds a significant sense of pressure to his erect penis, making it feel tighter, more engorged, and generally invincible.

If you're using a nonadjustable penis ring, put it on when your partner is soft; you can use adjustable straps at any point during an erection. Use some lube around the inside of the ring and on your partner's genitals to help place it around his penis or under his testicles and to avoid pulling his pubic hair (ouch!).

Once your man's erection is at high tide, his penis and/ or testicles will feel ultrasensitive. If the ring vibrates, waves of pleasure will wash over his entire groin region. In addition, your touches, licks, sucks, and strokes will be all the more intense, so go slowly at first to let him get used to it and enjoy it to the fullest. Start with light fondling around the perineum and testicles, then move up the shaft to brush against the head of his penis. Don't rush it; a penis ring can help delay ejaculation, so work with it.

If you're going to perform fellatio, start with lazy licks and delicate sucks until your partner asks you to go harder. If you're going to use your hands, warm some lube between your palms and then gently stroke his shaft with upward-only fingertip strokes before fist-pumping him up and down. And be sure to openly admire his gorgeous girth as you work on him. His penis may look larger than usual, so caress him with compliments too.

Of course, penis rings can also be used during intercourse. To increase your own pleasure, invest in a vibrating ring that is designed to stimulate a woman's clitoris during lovemaking. These have great erotic appeal and add significant sensation for both partners during sex. Have your partner vary the speed and angle of his thrusts until you find the combination that maximizes the ring's vibrating effect. Many men report that ejaculation and orgasm are intensified by the increased pressure the penis ring provides, so hold on tight as he climaxes.

A final word about penis rings: If your partner has never used one before, don't leave it on too long—probably not more than several minutes—and don't put it on too tightly. A misused ring can cause serious damage. Like any new toy, go slow and steady until you get the hang of it. If your partner experiences any pain whatsoever, remove the ring immediately. Adjustable straps are great for beginners, since they can be quickly and easily removed at the first sign of discomfort. The last thing you need is a two A.M. trip to the emergency room to have his new solid-steel cock ring sawed off by a troop of lip-biting nurses trying to avoid eye contact.

As most women know, men are visually stimulated. Many men are highly aroused by the sight of their partner in the throes of ecstasy, so your sex toolbox should contain a few female-friendly toys with which to give him a sexy show. Don't underestimate the power of girl gadgets, since they're often as or more enticing to men than male toys. Who knows, maybe they bring out the voyeur in them. Nipple clamps (they're not all as painful as they sound!) clip on to your nipples to create both a tingling effect for

You may want to avoid oil-based lubricants, such as petroleum jelly and baby oil, since their chemicals can break down condoms and sex toys. Oil-based lubes don't wash away as well as their water-based counterparts either, and can leave a coating on the vagina or rectum that can increase your chance of infection.

you and an erotic visual for your man. If you're having intercourse in the girl-on-top position, he can look up to watch your breasts bounce as never before. Some nipple clamps come with a chain, others with tassels, and still others vibrate. He won't be able to take his eyes off of you.

To move beyond mere appearances, consider including a dildo or strap-on dildo in your toolbox. Some men are very turned on by using these on their woman and/or by watching their woman pleasure herself with them. Let him penetrate you with a dildo or fasten a strap-on one around his thigh, and let him lie back and watch you lower yourself onto it to masturbate. To really set his bad-boy side free, ask him to use the head of the dildo to stimulate your anus. You don't have to put it inside since just the idea of fondling you in this way will spike his arousal. As with all sex toys, dildos come in as many shapes, sizes, textures, colors, material, and appearances as you can imagine.

Novelty condoms also have appeal to both men and women, and they too come in a host of colors, textures, scents, and flavors. If you're regular condom users, why not tuck those standard-issue drugstore rubbers into the back of your sock drawer now and then, and surprise your man by using something with more flair. He can watch as his bumpy blue neon manhood thrusts into you. If you and your partner don't normally use condoms, slide one onto him once in a while, just for a change. You don't have to keep it on for your whole session. Use it in foreplay by sliding it over his penis and performing fellatio (use a flavored condom if you like) so he can watch himself being sucked in a different way. You can always remove it when you want to get back to nature.

> Silicone-based lubes are the longest lasting and will stay slippery even underwater. They're good to use with latex condoms or toys but may degrade silicone sex toys. They're also a little harder to wash off than water-based lubes, but if you add a bit more soap they'll disappear down the drain.

Sweet treats are another fun item to include. Of course, there are the classic edible panties, but other options are far sexier. For example, there are some deliciously alluring body dusts, paints, and gels that smell as exquisite as they taste. You can let him watch while you spread them over your body, then let him lick them off. Or, cover his body with them and give yourself a sugar rush. As an appetizer, there's nothing sexier than a bite of rich dark chocolate to awaken the senses.

While not technically sex toys, adult videos and magazines are very effective erotic aids, and they are immensely useful when it comes to maintenance sex. For those times you want to pleasure your man but don't have the energy to bring him to full arousal, pop in a skin flick and let the pros do the work for you. Your man can lie down on the bed or sit back on the couch and watch the screen while you perform fellatio or give him a hand job. For many a man, this is pure sexual bliss. Watching pornography while his own woman pleasures him is like a big, juicy bite of forbidden fruit. He'll love the taste. Adult magazines are similarly useful, though somewhat less intense.

If you want to venture into more adventurous territory, see how your man responds to a penis pump. This is a popular male masturbation toy that delivers a wonderful suction sensation to a man's penis. To use, insert your partner's penis into the cylinder and use the hand pump to create a vacuum inside the cylinder. Having you work on his manhood in this way, particularly with this type of tool, may be a very sexually compelling experience for your man. Although they're fantastic solely for pleasure purposes, penis pumps are sometimes used to temporarily increase the size of the penis, and the fact that your man may briefly appear larger after use may be a bonus turn-on for both of you.

Okay. Sit tight. It's time to talk about anal play. Notice we didn't say anal *sex;* we just said anal *play.* This taboo territory has real erotic potential for men and women, but it isn't necessary to engage in anal intercourse or to insert an enormous dildo to enjoy what this playground has to offer. As we suggested earlier, the mere idea of stimulating a woman in this way may be enough to excite your man. But

> **Are you the sensitive type? If you've purchased a new type of lube, put a dab on the inside of your arm and wait a day to see if there's any reaction before using it in more southern climes.**

he too can enjoy the sensations the anal region can provide without the experience becoming too invasive, at least not in the beginning.

For many men, anal play is associated with homosexuality and therefore strictly off-limits. If you want to explore anal play or anal sex with your partner, you may first have to reassure him that the pleasurable experiences he feels "back there" do not mean he's gay. The pleasure comes from biology, not sexual orientation. Just as a woman's G-spot is stimulated via her vagina, a man's prostate is stimulated via the anus, and it's every bit as pleasurable to find. Once he's convinced of that fact, he may be more receptive to the idea, but don't expect too much; this is a squirmy issue for many people, particularly straight men. If your man doesn't want to do it, don't push the issue. Now that he knows you're game, he might surprise you and bring up the topic again after he's had some time to think about it.

If your man is willing to explore anal play, start off slowly by simply touching his anal region or inserting the tip of a well-lubed finger. Tell him not to worry about becoming aroused but simply to experience the sensations so he can become familiar with them and learn to relax.

Eventually, you should be able to insert more of your finger. The prostate is located a couple of inches in, toward the front of his body—turn your palm upward and curl your finger as if calling someone over.

When your man is ready to graduate from your finger to a full-fledged anal toy, consider starting with anal beads. Because they're less intimidating than a butt plug and less phallic than a dildo, he may be more willing to experiment with them. A string that offers graduated beads—small to larger—is best for beginners. Make sure that each bead is well-coated with a good-quality lubricant and ask your man to exhale and relax as you gently push the first bead into his anus. Follow his cues: if he wants you to insert more or larger beads, do as he wishes.

Once the beads are in place, it's more or less business as usual and you can turn your attention back to your man's penis. Regardless of how you pleasure him (whether via fellatio, hand job, or intercourse) the way in which you use the anal beads will depend on your partner's preferences. Some men like the beads to remain in place as they reach orgasm, while others like the string to be removed at the same time that they climax. Part of the fun is finding out.

Now that you're a fully certified sex toy specialist, tuck

> **Always, always, always use lots of lube during anal play.** There are thicker water- or silicone-based lubricants formulated specifically for anal sex, and some even include a desensitizer as an ingredient.

your tool box away, but make sure your partner knows where to find it and give him permission to pull it out whenever he feels that he's in need of a tune-up. You can even let him pick and choose which tool he'd like you to service him with. An on-demand, strictly maintenance lube job is one of the best ways to keep your man sexually satisfied. It's also a great way to ensure your relationship doesn't inadvertently spend too much time on cruise control.

Lube Job #12

●

Leather Seats

It wasn't as bad as I thought it would be. The strippers were pretty but not supermodel gorgeous, and Conner spent as much time checking the score on the big screen as he did staring at the dancers." Such is the confession of a peeler-bar initiate, Trina, a thirty-four-year-old wife of five years and mother of a ten-month-old baby.

"Curiosity made me go," Trina says. "The whole stripper-club scene is a subculture I'd never had any exposure to. I probably never would've gone just with Conner, but friends of ours told us they'd been going and invited us. That made it okay, since those wives were going. Safety in numbers."

"It felt really weird having Trina there," says her husband, Connor, thirty-four. "It felt like I shouldn't be looking. She kept whispering it was okay, and once she even whispered that it turned her on to watch me looking at the girls. That made it a lot easier. Then it seemed like we were doing it as a couple, and I didn't feel guilty. It was just fooling around, like foreplay."

"I don't know if I'd go again," Trina admits. "Maybe I would, but not for quite a while. It's a little too up close and personal for me. I think that kind of arousal should happen between two people in privacy, no third parties. I'm glad I went just so I know what it's like, but I don't think I'd want to make a habit out of it or use it as our regular form of entertainment. I prefer dinner and a movie. We did have fantastic sex when we got home, though."

Women do all sorts of things to add sizzle to their sex lives and arouse their men. Watching pornography, reading erotica, role playing, sporting new lingerie, using sex toys, and buying books like this are common efforts. Frequenting strip clubs may not be as popular a choice, but it's certainly nothing new, and many couples make the peelers a regular part of their sex life.

"My husband and I go at least once a month," says Trina's friend Jessie, thirty-six. "I find it erotic to watch the girls move, and the whole atmosphere is really charged with sex. I'm not attracted to the women in a sexual way, but watching them take off their clothes always gets me in the mood to do the same thing. They always look so sexy."

> Pole-dancing classes are the latest craze, but they aren't without controversy. Advocates say they can help a woman gain confidence and sensuality, while critics say they're just another way for a woman to please a man.

But what about jealousy?

"The strippers are just eye candy," Jessie insists. "I'd be more jealous if my husband were at the bar flirting with some drunken tart trying to get into his jeans. There'd be way more chance of cheating then. We have a 'look but don't touch' rule, and that works for us. People have different comfort levels and ideas about what constitutes cheating, but I don't think looking is cheating. A man is going to look no matter what, no matter where. You might as well be with him so you know what he's looking at. Anyway, it can have its advantages. My husband is the wildest lover whenever we get back from a strip club. It lights up his libido like the Fourth of July."

Other couples reserve the feather boas for special occasions only.

"My wife and I go once a year on my birthday," says Jonathan, thirty-two. "I don't care to go otherwise. It doesn't do much for me if I'm there with the guys, but it's fun to go with Lisa. It's good to do erotic things outside the bedroom so your sex life doesn't get in a rut, and that's why couples go to the clubs. It's different watching strippers than porn because it's right there in real time, but what turns me on most is the outfits the girls wear, all that leather and lace. I'm more turned on when they're dressed or partially dressed. My wife knows that, which is why my birthday gift always includes some skimpy new thing she's bought for herself. I know I'm going to see it when I get home, and I look forward to it all night. Great anticipation. I get to have stripper sex with my wife."

"It's all part of the seduction process," explains Lisa, thirty-five, Jonathan's wife of five years. "Men are visually aroused. They see a woman in a sexy outfit and wonder what she looks like naked, and that whole process turns them on. It's part of the chase. I like it when Jon watches the girls peel it off, because I know he's wondering what frilly teddy or lace bra is waiting for him at home. He likes it so much that I leave it on during sex."

Still not comfortable with your man being entertained by the sultry gyrations in a gentleman's club? You're not alone, and your discomfort doesn't mean you're insecure or prudish. It just means that, like Trina, you don't want to subcontract that side of your sex life. But there's more than one way to achieve this type of arousal and to let your man experience a voyeuristic sense of "the chase." For example, you can tap into the raw excitement of a one-night stand by parking outside a bar on a Saturday night, just before closing, and doing some mischievous people watching. As couples leave together, you can imagine how they hooked up inside, what he said to proposition her (or vice versa), where they're going, and what they'll do when they get there. The fiction you create together can be great foreplay and can give your partner a flashback feel of the chase. It's harmless two-person fun. Or, park in front of a seedy hotel—the charge-by-the-hour kind—and study the people coming and going, imagining the illicit affairs going on within. Play voyeur and pretend it's the two of you hooking up for a half-hour romp. As Jonathan pointed out, doing erotic things outside the bedroom is a good way to ensure your sex life doesn't fall into a rut of predictability, routine, and complacency.

When you get home from your voyeuristic wanderings, wherever they may have led you, the seduction process can really begin. Think you need a pole and a black vinyl bra-and-panty policewoman's uniform to seduce your man? Think again. There's a world of gorgeous lingerie out there that will make you feel as *femme fatale* as you look.

Too often, women look at the covers of lingerie catalogues and think, What's the point? I don't have that kind of body. The fact is, you don't need that kind of body to seduce your man. All you need is a new razor blade, a moisturizer, a splash of good perfume, and a sexy something to wear. Women know that men are visually aroused, yet it's astounding how many of us let our partners see us with leg hair thicker than the trees at Yosemite and dressed in clothes we wouldn't send our kids to the playground in.

Sure, we all have days where we want to slum in our sweatpants, but don't make it a habit. Here's a thought: use the buddy system. My sister and I have a brutally honest arrangement that keeps us in check. If I notice she's been remiss in her plucking duties and her cursed monobrow is silently closing in on her, I hand her the tweezers. If she's suddenly blinded by my gray roots reflecting the sun, she suggests I dial my stylist. It's easy to slack off, and sometimes it helps to have an honest compatriot sound the alarm. Women need maintenance, too, so keep your body feminine.

When you're plucked, shaved, scented, and soft, prepare to ice the cake with some lingerie before you offer your man a slice. When you dress for sex, your partner feels desired as a man, and he sees you as a woman, not just his wife or the mother of his kids. Sexy lingerie shouldn't be just for those long romantic evenings; it's a must for regular maintenance sex too. If a man is given two op-

Is your skin so white that it glows in the dark? For a healthy, year-round summer glow, use a moisturizer that comes with a skin-darkening complex. These are less dramatic than self-tanners, since the glow develops over several days. The hint of color will even out skin tone and make your skin look firmer, thereby increasing your confidence down the catwalk.

tions, (a) be pleasured by a woman in an old T-shirt and worn slippers or (b) be pleasured by a woman in a lace shelf bra and high heels, which route do you think most guys would prefer to travel? Our breasts, curves, hips, and legs are powerful tools with which to please our men, so put them to maximum use when performing maintenance sex.

Lingerie is available almost anywhere, from major department stores to specialty boutiques, and even racier, stripper-approved items can be found online. Plus-size shops carry equally erotic items, so there's a size and style to suit everyone. If you don't have a respectable drawerful of saucy wares from which to draw—for shame!—hit the shops before sundown. Don't waste another night waiting to lose those extra pounds or lamenting the gravitational forces at work on your breasts. Use what you have and find something that flatters your figure.

The classic baby doll is a good option for many figures as it comes in all styles, fabrics, and fashions. Go red-hot for a vixen look, virgin white for innocence incarnate, or black for bad-girl sophisticate. Bra-and-panty sets come in more cuts than you can count and are ideal for women who need breast support. Shelf bras are the she-devil's cut of choice since they lift the breasts from underneath but don't cover them up—talk about titillating! Push-up bras create voluptuous cleavage, and strapless bras are very enticing. Open-cup bras (a sexy version of the nursing bra) allow you to shamelessly flaunt your stuff, second only to the infamous nipple covers so often jostled about in peeler clubs.

Select a panty that similarly complements your body type. There are skirt-type panties for those thigh haters out there as well as low-rising/high-riding panties for those whose best assets are their buttocks. Boy-style panties are very cute, as are the traditional bikini-cut panties. Thongs are always popular (for those of us who can resist tugging, that is) and open-crotch panties are as carnal as they come.

Choose a matching bra-and-panty set with ruffles or lace to go ultrafeminine and pull on a pair of thigh-high stockings, preferably with a garter belt to combine the perfect amounts of vamp and class. Other options include snug bustiers and corsets, which also can be used with stockings and garters. Oh, yeah, don't forget to toss those churchgoing pumps and slip into a pair of shiny black high heels to complete the look of lust.

Finally, don't be in a hurry to lose the erotic effect of your lingerie. Since men are so visual, why not do what Lisa does and remain at least partially dressed during lovemaking? Crotchless panties make penetration easy, but any pair can be pushed to the side to allow entry, and the sight of his penis disappearing into your panties can be a salacious show for both of you. You can also wrap your legs

Depending on the style of lingerie you've chosen, you may want to accessorize with body jewelry. Waist chains are very alluring, and chokers are classic minx attire. A string of thick pearls or beads can serve a dual function: wrap them around your partner's penis and use them to stimulate him as he admires your barely clad body.

around him, still dressed in fishnets and heels, to accentuate an otherwise bare body and let him feel the sexy fabric against his skin.

Remember, clothes might make a man, but lingerie makes a woman. Dress for sex this evening, whether it's maintenance night or not, and give your visual man a real eyeful.

Lube Job #13

●

Zero Visibility

Now that we've spent the last chapter urging you to visually arouse your man, we're going to spend this one telling you to close his eyes. When sight is restricted, other senses become more acute: touches feel more exciting, caresses more consuming, and orgasms surprisingly intense. A blindfold may therefore be one of the most powerful and useful sexual aides you can employ. Add sex toys to a sightless sexual experience, and the body buzz can be electrifying.

While any toy can be used in a blindfolded sex session, the simple straight vibrator is one of the most versatile and

Use a sexy stocking with a spritz of perfume on it to blindfold your man. Stockings are great for restraints, too, unless you prefer the harder touch of handcuffs.

can bring a real charge to maintenance sex. If you're look-ing for an easy way to grease your guy's gears without actu-ally having to climb underneath the vehicle, you can use a vibrator on his genitals during a hand job or blow job for dramatic results.

Wrap the blindfold around your man's eyes, kiss him deeply on the mouth, and then ask him to lie back on the bed while you apply some personal lubricant to the vibra-tor and his genitals. Turn the vibrator on low and lightly roll it over his scrotum, then up his shaft and over the head of his penis. Slide it back down and hold it under his scro-tum so that it presses against his perineum. Check with him to make sure the vibration is at a pleasurable level, then hold the vibrator in place against his perineum with one hand while you stroke his penis to orgasm with the other hand.

If you're performing fellatio, you may wish to use your own saliva rather than a lubricant. In that case, use your mouth to slick up your man's genitals before you touch him with the vibrator. Move the vibrator in the same fashion—

> **When your man is lying back on the bed, occasionally shift the position of his legs while you use the vibrator on his penis and testicles. Have him lie with his legs straight together, then spread apart, and then knees bent. By changing the position of his legs, you can subtly affect the way the vibrations feel on his genitals.**

over his balls, up and down his shaft, over the head of his penis—as you lick and suck him with your mouth. Again, hold the vibrator against his perineum as you stroke and suck him to climax. Your mouth, the vibrator, and the blindfold will work together to give your guy an exquisitely erotic orgasm. If your partner likes to have his anus stimulated, you can also press the vibrator against this sensitive spot as you suck or stroke him.

To use the vibrator during intercourse, get in the woman-on-top position. Remember: it's maintenance sex, so you're doing the work tonight. When he's inside you, slip the vibrator between your bodies so it touches your clitoris. Once you've done this, you may find the experience goes from maintenance to mutual. Reach around and roll the vibrator over his balls and under his scrotum, again stimulating his perineum with deeply felt vibrations that may reach all the way to his prostate. Pump his penis with your body as you, the blindfold, and the vibrator bring him to a body-shuddering orgasm. What a ménage à trois!

To add another guest to the party, you can use restraints to really keep your man in his place. Helena, twenty-seven, found that restraints helped her to overcome her main obstacle to effective maintenance sex.

"My problem would've made most women jealous," Helena admits. "I found it difficult to do maintenance sex on my boyfriend because he wouldn't let me. He's a very sensitive lover, very considerate, but there are times when a woman just doesn't want to have sex no matter how good her lover is. I still wanted to satisfy him during those times, but he was so preoccupied with pleasing me that he wouldn't ever relax and just receive pleasure. It sounds silly

You can also perform this lube job while your man sits on a chair. Bind his arms to the armrests and his legs to the legs of the chair. He's now in the perfect position to feel your mouth, hands, and the vibrator work their wonders on his groin.

but that can be frustrating, especially since I sometimes had to fake an orgasm just so he'd let me do my part."

Okay, you don't have to share Helena's attitude, but her frustration was as real as her solution was effective.

"I was trying to give him a hand job one night, but he kept pushing my hands away and kissing my nipples and what not, trying to arouse me. The harder he tried, the more irritated I became because I just wanted to satisfy him and go to sleep. I wasn't interested in sex. Then I had a revelation. His tie was on the floor, so I rolled over to grab it, then tied his wrists to the bedposts like I was a pro. His jaw dropped, but he didn't stop me. I told him that he was at my mercy and I was going to make him come my way. It solved the problem. He was turned on, his hands didn't roam, and it was all over in about ten minutes. He thought I was being sexy, but I was being practical."

Now that's maintenance sex done right.

To keep the use of restraints exciting, wrap the blindfold around your man's eyes while he's tied up. You can also tie his ankles to the footboard. When he's bound and blindfolded, use the vibrator to stimulate his genitals as you alternate between hand and oral pleasure. His groin

Blindfolds and restraints are the very softest side of S&M (sadomasochism) and sexual acts of domination and submission. Want to go a little further? Try dripping hot wax on your partner's bare skin to really heat things up. Erotic hot-wax candles can be purchased at sex shops: Be sure to educate yourself on the proper type of candles and their use, lest your burning lust become a third-degree burn.

should be a hot spot of vibrating, sucking, and stroking sensations. Make him come at your whim, or climb on top and finish with woman-on-top intercourse. Whatever way you bring him to orgasm, he won't see it coming.

Lube Job #14

●

The Fast and the Furious

Long sleeves, short sleeves, three-quarter-length sleeves—your closet probably has them all, but for this lube job, you'll need a sleeve of a very different sort in your closet: a penis sleeve. In case you've never seen one, a penis sleeve is a sex toy for men, a type of artificial vagina (or anus or even mouth) that is available in a host of sizes, shapes, and styles. Some even vibrate. But whether it's battery powered or not, a penis sleeve is the right tool for this fast and furious lube job, and an accessory that no closet should be without.

Penis sleeves are a favorite male masturbation toy that you won't have any trouble finding at any sex shop. The better models boast natural-feeling materials and various textures to heighten sensation during thrusting. They're also adjustable to increase the suction and friction on a man's penis. Because there are so many brands and options available, shop around until you find the one you think would arouse your partner the most. And don't forget to pick up some water-based lubricant to use with your new purchase.

Since you'll ultimately be using the penis sleeve in the dark, you'll want to acquaint yourself with its shape and where it will require lubrication. When action is imminent, you'll be squirting some of the lube inside the sleeve itself as well as lubricating the opening through which your partner's penis will pass, so you may want to do a dry run just for practice.

Now that your toolbox is equipped and you're ready to perform some regular maintenance on your man, choose a

> **Penis sleeves are sometimes used as practice for the real thing—you! Some men find this type of sex toy is a good tool to fine-tune their ejaculation control.**

suitable location. A spacious closet is best, although any dark, enclosed nook will do. To avoid mattress monotony, it's wise to surprise your man with a quickie outside of the bedroom whenever possible. Lube jobs often exploit the exciting unfamiliarity of a spontaneous sexual encounter beyond the bedroom walls, and this racy closet quickie may be the best of the bunch.

The timing of this quickie is entirely up to you. You can perform it just before bed, in the middle of a lazy weekend afternoon, or the moment your man gets home from work. Stash the penis sleeve and lube under the linens in your closet, and you'll be prepared for action anytime you please. Just make sure your mother-in-law isn't staying over, or you'll have questions to answer when she reaches in for a bath towel.

When you're ready to tune up your man, lead him with a wink into the closet and close the doors. Make up a sexy story to tell him as you undress the both of you. For example, tell him that he's at a party when you, a seductive stranger, take him by the hand and lead him into a dark, hidden closet. You undress yourself and him, and then take his hands and run them all over your body, over the mounds of your breasts and hard nipples, down to the slippery softness between your legs. You reach down to squeeze his cock, gasping at how hard and thick it is. Finally, you turn your back to him and press your ass against his groin. Desperate, you beg him to enter you . . . from behind.

Sure, this is dirty talk, but your goal is to make your partner as hard as possible as fast as possible, so don't waste time reciting love poetry. If you really want to rev his engine and if you think your partner would be game, tell him the stranger wants to have anal sex. This will be particularly arousing if you and your partner don't normally practice anal play; simply toying with the idea of a taboo activity can be a great way to experience escapist sex and forbidden fun.

Move your man's hands over your body and between your legs. Tell him how good it feels to have him touch you, then reach out and caress his body and genitals ever so lightly. When he's hard, retrieve the lube and penis sleeve. He'll know you're up to something, but don't tell. Let him guess in the dark. Warm the lube in your palms and then spread it on your partner's penis. As you practiced, insert some lube into the sleeve and apply some to the opening.

Turn your back to your man and place the sleeve between your legs with the opening facing backward, toward him. Ask him to stand close behind your body and penetrate you. As he gets into position, reach around and slide his erect penis into the sleeve. Again, don't tell him what you're doing or using, just let him bask in the new sensations and wonder what you're up to. Tell him he's inside the sexy stranger, perhaps inside her "ass," and ask him to start thrusting. As he does, hold the sleeve as securely as you can between your legs, using your hands to hold it in place as his excitement grows and his thrusts intensify.

Remember that it's the diversity and unexpectedness of these quickies that will enrapture your man, not the flawless positioning of the penis sleeve or a Pulitzer-quality erotic story. Don't get caught up in perfect choreography. Just relax, hold on to the sleeve, and let your own storytelling unfold as you like. Take your cues from your partner. If you say something that makes him groan and grab your hips, elaborate. If you experience mechanical problems with the sleeve, laugh it off and begin again. Should the sleeve prove undoable, it's no big deal. Throw it to the floor and have your man thrust into your tight-fisted hands. Adapt, have fun with it, and nothing can go wrong.

There are several forces at work in this lube job that will likely compel your partner to reach orgasm with fast and furious intensity. The spontaneity of the encounter, the excitement of the unusual location, the standing rear-entry position, and the taboo idea of anal sex with a stranger, all combined with your dirty story, is a potent formula for a fantastic quickie.

Of course, the most powerful feature of this maintenance quickie is the innovative and unexpected use of a sexual aide. If you and your partner don't usually use toys, or at least not this type of toy, the surprise and novelty of the experience will be just as arousing to your man as the flood of new sensations the penis sleeve will provide. This lube job won't last long, so don't worry if dinner's in the oven. And, conveniently, you probably won't be too far from a towel for postquickie cleanup.

AMOROUS ANCESTORS
Upper Paleolithic art dating back 30,000 years depicts people using dildos to pleasure themselves and others. That means mankind invented sex toys long before the wheel. The time line speaks to our priorities, doesn't it?

As your man catches his breath, tuck the sleeve away at the back of the closet but not too far back. It might be back in fashion sooner than you think.

As we've said, variety is one of the most important ingredients in a good sex life. The inclusion of a few erotic toys in your sexual repertoire is an easy and effective way to add a new dimension to your lovemaking. To prove the popularity of sexual aides, notice the number of sex shops that have sprung up in all major (and not so major) urban centers. Sex toys, along with adult videos, are now in the mainstream, and the secrecy associated with purchasing these items is a thing of the past.

Nonetheless, if you're still hesitant about visiting a sex shop, here's an idea: before you go, do an Internet search for "sex toys" to familiarize yourself with the appearance and usage of some of these adult items. A little sex-toy education in the privacy afforded by your own computer may boost your confidence before you stroll down the sex aisles, eye level with the double-ended dildos and butt plugs. If you're still too uncomfortable to take that vibrating cock ring you really like to the counter, you can purchase it online and have it delivered to your door in a nice, safe, anonymous brown box. Your neighbors will never know what's inside. Unless their anal beads are being delivered the same day, that is.

One couple who would never dream of ordering their sex toys online is David and Amy. Together for seven years, one of their favorite foreplay pastimes is to visit the sex shop arm in arm and to take their sweet time browsing the inventory and choosing the perfect erotic accoutrement to their evening's planned festivities.

"We call it retail foreplay," says Amy. "We take our time walking up and down the rows, looking at all the different toys and pictures, and talking about what we'd like to use on each other. The whole process is a wicked aphrodisiac."

"We're so turned on by the time we get home," adds David, "that we barely have time to insert the batteries before we're clambering to undress each other. It's very powerful."

According to David and Amy, the most crucial requirement of their particular love life is constant variety. They both admit to becoming quickly bored—that's just their nature—and they rely on the changing inventory of the sex shops they visit to prevent sexual predictability and routine from creeping into the bedroom.

"We do get bored quickly," explains Amy, "but it doesn't take much to get the spark back. Even experimenting with a new brand of lubricant or tasting a flavored whipping cream is enough to send us over the edge again. I guess we're lucky that way."

Fortunately, most couples don't get bored as readily or as often as David and Amy, but their tried-and-true approach to keeping their sex life dynamic and fulfilling works for them, and that's what matters. In fact, it's a blessing they've found each other and that they are both willing to do what it takes, together, to keep their relationship thriving. Their communication skills as a couple are exceptional, and they have a profound understanding of each other's sexual needs and desires.

> Watch your body language. Nonverbal messages are a powerful part of a couple's communication. Be aware of the signals you're sending your partner and keep them positive. Make eye contact during conversation; smile when he comes in the room; and flirtatiously play with your hair when you look at him.

That understanding extends to maintenance. While Amy is sated by her three-times-a-week average, she says that her man runs most smoothly on five or even six times a week. She proudly admits that maintenance sex is especially easy for her to perform since she already has a toolbox with enough toys to stock any sex superstore to the rafters. Equipped with this arsenal of sexual aides—from penis pumps to fingertip vibrators—she is able to keep her sexually driven but easily bored partner more than satisfied.

"I make sure that I don't rely too much on one thing for too long," says Amy. "If David's really into it for a long stretch, I alternate the toys I use on him. One day I'll use the pump. Another day I'll use a vibrator while I suck him off."

"I never know what she's going to pull on me," David reveals, "especially after we've been to one of those sex trade shows that come around every couple of years. Those are total windfalls for me. I give her the credit card, a big brown bag, and tell her to put us in as much debt as she wants to. Money can buy some kinds of happiness, you know."

As we've said, and as Amy and David obviously recognize, variety is one of the most important features of a healthy and happy love life. It is equally important when it comes to the specific issue of maintenance sex. Just as Amy has done, you should strive to pleasure your man in new ways when his sex drive slips into overdrive. So the next time you and he pass one of those neon-lit sex shops, why not take a quick detour inside to see what they might have in store for you?

Lube Job #15

○

Remote-Controlled Pleasure

Did you ever see someone yawn and then yawn yourself? It's contagious. I'm yawning just thinking about it, and you might be too. Well, wake up; I'm trying to make a point, not send you off for a siesta. Feelings can also be contagious, and this is especially true when it comes to sexual arousal. A low moan from the downstairs apartment or the neighboring hotel room can often be more of a turn-on than the graphic sight of frantic porno pumping. The sights and sounds of another person's arousal can be a powerful aphrodisiac, and we'll be putting that fact to good use in this lube job. We'll also be putting to use another accessory from your sex toolbox—a remote-controlled bullet vibrator.

As with most sex toys, there are infinite variations of the bullet vibrator, sometimes called a vibrating egg massager. The bullet is inserted into the vagina, and its type and speed of vibration is adjusted via a remote control. The bullets can be of varying shapes and sizes, and some units even come with interchangeable bullets. Cordless models are widely available, and the number, speed, and variety of pulse settings also vary from model to model. You'll also want to ensure that the unit you select has a good range and low volume.

The next time you're getting dolled up for date night, insert the bullet vibrator before you pull on your pantyhose. Sometime during the evening, perhaps right after dinner, pass the remote control to your partner and enlighten him on its features. Tell him he's at the wheel. Close your eyes in ecstasy and moan under your breath whenever your partner exercises his control over your pleasure. Circle your hips and lick your lips to let him enjoy the sounds and sights of your arousal, thereby becoming aroused himself. Don't be surprised if he wants to head home before the dessert menu arrives.

Remote-control panties are an all-in-one alternative to an internal bullet vibrator. The vibrator is built into the panty itself and therefore stays outside the body, providing vibrations to the clitoris and outer vagina.

When you're back in your bedroom, tell your man to stay at the controls while you undress. Let him watch you peel off your clothes as he randomly sends pulses and waves of pleasure through your body. Whew! Your man's heart will be pounding, and his other body parts will be too. When you're naked, lie back on the bed as he continues to manipulate your body. Not only will the visual of seeing your body in this way turn him on, but his sense of the sexual power he has over you will also ignite his desire.

Ask him to undress, then have him join you on the bed and touch your naked, writhing body as the bullet pulses inside you. You want your man to lose himself in the erotic control he has over your body. When you're ready, have him get into whatever position he'd like to receive fellatio in, whether it's lying on his back, kneeling, sitting, or standing. Give him oral pleasure as he continues to stimulate you via remote control. No doubt the two of you will find your own rhythm: perhaps the more pulses he delivers to you, the harder you suck on him.

It's up to you and your partner whether you bring him to orgasm with fellatio or whether you want to move on to intercourse. If you do want to have intercourse, remove the bullet and let your partner watch as you tease your clitoris and nipples with its vibrations—with his fingers on the dial, of course. When your partner finally penetrates you (the good ol' missionary position is great for this), slip the bullet between your bodies so that it will continue to stimulate your clitoris as he thrusts. You'll both feel the vibrations, and many women find they achieve very intense orgasms this way. Make sure the remote control is at your partner's fingertips at all times so that he can play with the controls as he wishes, thereby changing the pulsations you both feel during sex.

This red-hot lube job is a devilishly fun way to recharge the batteries in your love life. Its eroticism comes in part from sexual contagion, since the more aroused your partner sees you, the more aroused he becomes. But the erotic charge in this lube job also comes from something else: the sense that he has control—sexual power—over you, even if it's only make-believe.

Nowadays, there are precious few places where a man can still exercise his primal masculinity and control. Let's face it. Women have had to fight tooth and nail to sit in the driver's seat, and we're sometimes reluctant to slide into the passenger's seat and let someone else take the wheel, particularly if that someone else is a man. This lube job is therefore a great vehicle for letting your partner play with a sense of power. Let him hold the controls once in a while; he'll feel powerful, and you'll be pampered.

Power struggles are common in relationships, and regardless of how they begin or what fuels them, they inevitably find a way to slip under the bedroom door and cause problems in a couple's sex life. But by being aware of and addressing the power issues in your relationship, you can prevent this tug-of-war from sneaking under the bed sheets.

The power struggle between Meredith and Ben, a married couple with two preschool-age children, illustrates a power issue that is increasingly common in this world of the successful working woman. For the first four years of their marriage, Meredith worked from home as a freelance graphic artist, making a modest salary that did not compare to Ben's high-salary position as foreman at a large commercial construction company. Although her career wasn't as successful as she imagined it would be, her ability to work from home nevertheless gave Meredith the opportunity to stay at home with her children, which she had wanted to do. All in all, the arrangement was working well . . . until the downsizing, that is.

It was a regular Monday morning when Ben discovered that his employer had sold the construction company and that his high-paid position did not fit into the plans the new owners had for the company. By noon he was back home with a severance package in his hand and a sinking feeling in his stomach. He and Meredith needed a new plan, and they needed it fast. They both began job hunting, and they were both surprised when Meredith struck career gold first. Within two weeks they had switched places: Meredith was a working mom, and Ben was a stay-at-home dad.

"It was a dream job," says Meredith. "My university degree was paying off; my time in the freelance trenches was paying off; and I had the job I had dreamed of for years. It happened suddenly, but I was ready to do it. The kids were a little older, out of diapers at least, and I was starting to miss working outside the home. Plus, I knew Ben could handle the kids. He's always been a great dad."

"It was a classic case of seemed-like-a-good-idea-at-the-time," says Ben. "The first few months were great. I didn't have to race out of the house at six A.M., I didn't have to take calls through every meal, and I didn't have the stress of big-buck jobs hanging over my head. The kids were awesome. We had lots of fun and did all kinds of things together: swimming, bicycling, flying kites in the park, you name it. I was a glossy poster for the fulfilled, well-adjusted stay-at-home dad."

But how did this construction foreman turned domestic figurehead handle the household duties of cooking and cleaning?

"He's a better dad than housewife," jokes Meredith. "The kids had never been happier—everyday they did something different—but the house, frankly, went to hell. I'd come home at six o'clock, and supper would be spilling out of pots on the stove. The table was never set. The laundry waited until the weekend, when I did it, and I don't think the bathtub was scrubbed for a month. Sometimes, as a hint, I'd take the vacuum out before I left for work in the morning, but it would still be standing in the same place when I got home. The floor was still crunchy. He didn't seem to do any cleaning at all, and that really got on my nerves. I hated coming home to a dirty house day after day."

Eventually, Meredith's silent irritation with Ben's lax housekeeping turned into vocal frustration. If she came home to a sink full of dishes, she'd sigh loudly and remind him that she had managed to both clean the house and care for the children. If the kids were wearing mismatched clothing, she'd shake her head at his fashion faux pas. And if Ben bought something, whether a new pair of shoes for the kids or a small television for his weight room, she'd raise her eyebrows and ask how much it cost.

"Meredith did get a touch of the queen bee syndrome," says Ben. "I can understand it, since she'd spent many years struggling to get her career off the ground. Then she got this dream job, and for the first time in her life was making really good money and actually getting the recognition she deserved. But I can't say she didn't start to treat me a bit like a drone. Our sex life slowed to a crawl, and I felt like she'd only give me sex when I'd performed everything up to her specs. Worst of all, I started to feel like a kept man, a financial dependent. That doesn't exactly fire up a man's libido."

> Be careful what you wish for. When a drone (a male honeybee) finally mates with a queen bee, its abdomen is ripped open during copulation, and it dies soon afterward.

"He's right, I was the queen bee for a while," Meredith admits. "Ben had never questioned me on the cost of things I'd buy for myself or the kids, but I'd grill him. And he knew I wouldn't have sex unless things were done around the house. Our love life definitely started to go downhill. For the first time, I was the breadwinner, and I was keenly aware of that. I was going full-speed ahead in my career, and I was scared to slow down or I'd lose my position. It was all new to me, and I had a sense of power, including sexual power, which I wasn't above flaunting to Ben. I started to see my marriage almost as a parent-child relationship, and that obviously wasn't a turn-on for either of us."

While many arrangements involving working women and stay-at-home men are happy and successful, Meredith and Ben had a difficult time making the transition, largely because of Meredith's sudden rise to power. There's no doubt that women have fought to overcome economic, social, and political oppression, and that fight is far from over. In fact, the fight is deeply ingrained in both the modern woman's psyche and reality. Sadly, however, this battle often crosses the work field to invade the bedroom.

Women use skill, determination, and hard work to achieve equal power in the business and political arenas. Yet they often use sex to control the power balance in their personal relationships, where they sometimes strive for superiority rather than mere equality. Who knows, maybe they're unconsciously punishing their well-intentioned men for the sins of their suffrage-withholding forefathers. Regardless of the reason, when a woman uses sex as a power tool, as Meredith did, a couple's love life will suffer. Relationship repair comes with empathy and understanding. Once each partner is able to empathize with the other's struggles and understand the other's emotional needs, the damage can be reversed.

Women struggle with issues of unequal pay, chauvinistic employers, and the guilt-ridden boxing match between the stay-at-home and working-mother camps. Even today, women are often judged by their cup size rather than their credentials, and the pressure to have it all—successful career, perfect kids, handsome husband, great body—is always on. But just as society snubs the woman who doesn't "have it all," so does it demean the man who doesn't climb the ladder of institutional and financial success. Never mind that he's a devoted husband and loving father, what's his job title? How much did he make last year? This can be an emasculating culture for men. Just as popular culture belittles women who aren't a size two, it also marginalizes men who don't make a six-figure income.

"My queen bee days came to an end in an eye-opening

way," says Meredith. "Ben and I were lying in bed, and he was doing his best to initiate sex. I was peeved that he hadn't gotten groceries that day, so I ignored his advances and asked why he didn't go shopping. He told me he didn't have enough money in his wallet, and asked if I could leave him some tomorrow. I could tell he was humiliated."

"I felt like somebody had castrated me," continues Ben. "I wouldn't be surprised if I actually looked down to make sure my balls were still there."

Pussy whipped is a state all men dread. We might laugh at the term, but if we think about the meaning of the phrase—to be defeated, punished, controlled, conquered, dominated—it loses some of its humor. Improve your vocabulary and your relationship by focusing on the meaning of words like *support, praise, equality, love,* and *respect* instead.

"That obviously broke the mood," says Meredith. "I felt like his mother, giving him lunch money. And I can't even imagine how he must have felt."

"I felt like a loser," Ben clarifies, "and I did *not* feel like having sex."

"It didn't take more than that moment for me to understand how he had been feeling," says Meredith. "I could tell just by the look in his eyes. He'd always been an excellent provider, and, to be honest, I'd always been attracted to that. That part of his identity had been taken away, and

I began to realize just how much his sense of manhood was being threatened, especially since I'd been withholding sex. We didn't have sex that night either, but we did talk a lot about our insecurities and how we could support each other emotionally. I told him how scared I was to lose the job I had worked so hard for. I'd fought so long to be taken seriously that I had to focus on turning off my domineering 'boss' side when I got home."

"It was an excellent talk," says Ben. "Normally I can't stand to talk about my feelings and all that, but it felt good to get it off my chest. I told Meredith how difficult it is for a man who's always had a sense of control to hand over the reins. I told her that I loved being with the kids but that her complaints about the housework made me feel whipped. We talked a lot about how it was affecting our sex life, too. I still felt the urge to have sex, but, to be brutally honest, I was losing sexual attraction to her. She doled out sex like a miser doles out money, and I had to beg for it. I didn't feel like she needed or appreciated me, and that did affect how much I desired her."

"I concentrated on giving Ben a feeling of empowerment in his life and in his decision to stay home with the kids," Meredith explains, "which is something he'd always done for me when I was a stay-at-home mom. I left the queen bee at the office. At home, I was his wife and my kids' mother. I really had to work on keeping those roles separate at first, but it's easier now and we're both happier. I made him feel appreciated, and I showed him how much the kids and I needed him. As for the housework, we compromised and hired a cleaning service to come in twice a week. As for the sex, I made him feel like an irresistible stud in bed. I guess there's some wisdom to letting the man be on top once in a while!"

Maintenance sex is about more than dealing with disparate sex drives. It's also about maintaining the integrity of the intimate relationship as a whole, about recognizing the differences not only in the sexual needs between men and women but also in the emotional needs. Just as a woman longs to feel loved, secure, and beautiful in her man's eyes, a man longs to feel needed, powerful, and appreciated by his woman. If your man makes you feel emotions that fulfill you, why not return the favor?

> ### ✲ SIGNED, SEALED, DELIVERED
> Mail a thank-you card to your man at work, expressing your gratitude for all the things he does for you. Tell him the many reasons you're thankful for having him in your life. It's the male equivalent of a love letter and a dozen long-stemmed red roses.

While the remote-controlled bullet vibrator in this lube job is a fun way to give your man a playful sense of sexual control, be sure to remember that nonsexual feelings also affect his pleasure between the sheets. Whether he's a highly paid executive or an underappreciated worker bee, you have a great deal of control over how he feels about himself both inside and outside the bedroom. And if you fulfill his emotional needs as well as his sexual needs, you'll be the object of his affection as much as of his desire.

Part Four

Sexual
Intercourse

Lube Job #16

◉

Reading the Map—Written Erotica

Erotica, a word derived from the Greek *eros* (love), is a style of writing that is intended to evoke sexual desire. Generally speaking, erotica is more tame, tasteful, and egalitarian or female-friendly than written pornography, although the distinction between the two is often hazy. The erotica in this chapter is meant to appeal to an intelligent, mainstream readership who can use it as a sort of aphrodisiac or form of foreplay: by reading these erotic stories together, a couple can increase their sexual arousal in a fun, exciting, and nonthreatening way.

For some couples who do not watch adult movies, written erotica is an ideal alternative. Sandra and Bill, a young couple who found the sounds and vocalizations in adult movies to be nothing short of thigh-slappingly hilarious, weren't opposed to pornography in principle; in fact, they often enjoyed looking at pornographic magazines together. However, whenever they tried to watch a skin flick, the array of grunts and slaps and *ooh*s and *aah*s doubled them over with laughter. Turning down the volume didn't help. They soon became so preoccupied and distracted by even imagining what sounds were being made, that they simply couldn't separate the visual from the audio. For the time being at least, adult movies weren't destined to play a big part in their sex life.

Eventually, Sandra began to read aloud the erotic letters that were featured in their pornographic magazines. To their surprise, reading these letters often aroused them even more than looking at the images in the magazines or on-screen. As Bill explained, the arousal came from a combination of hearing the erotic words spoken by his girlfriend, being immersed in the alluring storyline, and using his imagination to flesh out the enticing details. It wasn't long before they graduated from amateur letters to quality published erotica.

> Written erotica comes in both fiction and nonfiction. If your literary tastes lean toward the voyeuristic, choose nonfiction to see what your neighbors have been up to. Some nonfiction erotica collections focus on a committed couple's sexual adventures together, which may be particularly appealing to readers.

Although both Sandra and Bill admitted that they would continue to view pornography and eventually try to watch adult films again, it is worth noting that both of them expressed feeling greater sexual intimacy and emotional connection while reading erotica together than they did while viewing pornographic material. This sentiment is echoed by many erotica lovers who find the fantasy worlds they explore together in books highly conducive to connecting not only sexually but also emotionally.

For those couples who either regularly or on occasion do enjoy adult films (including the grunts and slaps and *ooh*s and *aah*s), written erotica is a perfect way to add even more variety to their sexual repertoire. Erotica can enhance a couple's sexual experience by providing new ideas and bringing fantasy to lovemaking. Good erotica should be as escapist as it is arousing, allowing the mind to wander to forbidden and sexually exhilarating places, people, and possibilities.

> *Fanny Hill: Memoirs of a Woman of Pleasure* is widely considered to be the first erotic novel. Written by John Cleland in 1749, the novel was banned in the United States until 1966. And although it was for many years reviled as pornography, it's now considered a literary classic.

The three erotic stories we have included here are the ultimate in escapist erotica. They are also highly explicit and share a common plot element: an individual performing an intensely provocative sex dare as an initiation rite for membership in a secret sex society. Each sex dare is as erotically thrilling as it is taboo, and each initiate has an incredible story to tell following his or her particular challenge.

Although you will likely discover your own way to use these stories, many couples find that this type of written erotica is best used as foreplay to sexual intercourse, and we'd have to agree. Men and women find this material equally arousing, and once the storyline captures the sexual attention, there's nowhere to go but to the bedroom.

When it comes to maintenance sex, written erotica can be especially useful. A literary lube job is a fun and effortless way for a woman to increase her man's arousal without having to exert a lot of time or energy herself. We've all heard it said that the mind is the largest sexual organ, and there's a great deal of truth to that. These edgy stories will have your man's sexual imagination in overdrive in record-breaking time.

As a suggestion, try surprising your partner as he lies in the bath. Sit on the edge of the tub while he bathes and read him a story. By the time you're finished and he's clean, you'll both be ready to get dirty again. Or, hide under the bed covers and have some fun reading a dare together by flashlight. Once you've turned the last page and are ready to turn to each other, you won't have far to reach.

You can also combine this erotica with sensual massage, perhaps caressing your man while he reads to let him bask in both pleasures at once. Better yet, have him massage your body while you read a story to him. It's a win-win situation: he gets fantastic foreplay, and you get a free deep-muscle massage.

Regardless of how you perform these literary lube jobs, they offer effortless sexual foreplay at its finest and will

> **Want to give your eyes a break?** Give auditory erotica a try. Sexy CDs featuring erotic stories and the sounds of couples having sex are quickly gaining popularity. Slip one into your bedside CD player, snuggle next to your man, and press play. It's foreplay you can actually hear!

likely have you combing the bookstore shelves for the thickest volumes of erotica available. So, dog-ear this chapter and tuck this book under your pillow, and the next time you need an easy way to kick-start your man's motor, dare yourself—or him—to start reading.

The Truck Stop

Female, thirty
DES MOINES, IOWA

The chauffeur drove to the outskirts of town and then continued on to the highway. Eventually, we pulled into a huge twenty-four-hour truck stop. There was a digital clock in the limousine, and I remember that it was exactly 3:17 A.M. I had never been to one of those big truck stops before, the really sprawling kind, and when we drove around the building, I was amazed at the number of semis in the parking lot. There were rows and rows of them with all kinds of trailers and loads, most wearing out-of-state plates. Some were idling, but many were quiet.

The chauffeur drove up and down the rows slowly, and I looked out my window at the huge trucks as we passed by. Finally, the limousine stopped, and the driver turned around to face me, smiling as he revealed my dare: "There are prostitutes," he said, "called lot lizards. They go around to truck stops every night and offer sex to the drivers." He smiled wider and said, "Go." He handed me a pager, at least I think it was a pager, and told me to press the button if I needed help. He said he'd be close.

I got out of the limousine, and as soon as I stood on the pavement, the reality of what I was doing struck home. It was as though everything in the universe was waiting to see what I would do. The huge trucks looked so strange and daunting, especially in that weird haze that was somewhere between late night and early morning, and I felt like I was in an alien world. The still air, the moonlight reflecting off the chrome of the stacks and bumpers, and the twisting nervousness of my stomach all made me feel completely disconnected from my real life.

My footsteps echoed off the pavement of the quiet parking lot as I approached the first truck. It was red, with a really big sleeper on the back. Fueled by adrenaline and desire, I grabbed on to the handle and put my foot onto the metal step, then pulled myself up to peek inside the window. It was dark inside and hard to see. I held on to the handle with my right hand and tapped gently on the window. Nothing. I tapped again, louder.

I heard rustling from inside the truck and held my breath. I wondered what the guy would look like, what he'd do, and what I'd do. I was so scared he'd shout at me or somehow draw attention to me. My courage was coming from the fact that these trucks were from far away, and that I was—and would remain—a stranger. If somebody had drawn attention to me, I wouldn't have been able to handle it. I needed to stay anonymous.

Finally a face emerged from the sleeper and peered out the window at me. To my horror, it was a woman. She looked confused for a moment, then her expression changed to anger. I knew what she was mad about. She thought I was a hooker coming to hit on her husband or boyfriend, and she was pissed. I heard her yell through the glass, and I jumped down from the truck.

My heart was racing from embarrassment, yet I also felt empowered by the experience. It had gone badly but not as badly as it could have, and now I at least knew that I could do it. The very next truck, a blue one, looked a little older than the red one and was quite dirty. It looked like it had been on the road for a long time, which meant that the driver was from far away. I liked that. My hesitation was abating, and I was starting to see the whole thing as a challenge. I guess that's what it's supposed to be. To be honest, the uncertainty and the search for the right truck was the most potent foreplay I'd ever experienced. There was no guarantee I would succeed, and that made me want to all the more.

I climbed up the blue truck and tapped on the window. I instantly heard movement in the sleeper, and again I started to worry what the driver might look like. A man's face appeared at the window. He stared out blankly for a moment, then what I was doing there must have registered. He rolled down the window and smirked a hello.

I smiled as suggestively as I could. To be completely honest, it was easy since I found him attractive. He was a big man, not fat, just big: the type that can throw you around the bed, and I like that. He had a nice face, too. Not exactly handsome, but he was perfect for my purpose. I knew the second I saw him that he'd be willing. He didn't look weird or creepy or anything; he just looked like the type of hot-blooded guy who wouldn't turn down sex. I said, "I'm kinda new at this," and he replied, "Sure thing, kitten. New is good. We'll take it slow."

He asked me to get down so he could open the door, and I did. He pushed it open, and I climbed back up into the cab of the truck, slamming the door closed behind me. It was warm inside the cab, fairly clean, and smelled vaguely like lemon car freshener. He didn't ask me anything, but I felt compelled to volunteer something. I tried to jump into the role. I asked, "Have you been wanting some company tonight?" and he replied, "Yeah. I've been on the road a long time, so company would be real nice."

There was no doubt we both knew what was going to happen. The knowledge made me relax, and I started to enjoy it even more. The certainty that sex would happen and that we both wanted it was a relief. Now I could just soak in the thrill of it all. The hard part was over. I had forced myself to do something I never dreamed I could do, and now I was reaping the reward. Sex with a total stranger in a place I'd never even imagined. My whole body was on fire with anticipation: the buds of my hard nipples were pressing against my bra and my clit was already starting to swell.

The inside of the truck was not as cramped as I thought it would be. The guy, his name was Jack, asked me if I wanted to lie down in the back with him. He crawled into the sleeper, and I placed the pager on the dash before I followed him. He was dressed in jeans and a T-shirt. I don't know if he was sleeping in his clothes or had dressed when I knocked. Our bodies touched when we both climbed in the back, and I felt like my skin would burst into flames it was so hot. Jack asked me if I wanted to watch a movie, and I noticed he had a small television set in the sleeper. I knew it was just an excuse to get close, so I nodded and said yes.

He slipped a DVD in and turned on the TV. My stomach flipped when a porn flashed across the screen. It was an image of a woman's open legs with a man's hands roaming between them. I asked him if he kept this kind of movie with him all the time. He said, "All the time, honey. It gets lonely on the road. A man's got needs." He winked.

I thought about him watching these movies and masturbating back there by himself. I've always been turned on by the idea of a man stroking himself, and I imagined his rough, callused hands sliding over the smoothness of his cock. I felt like I was being pumped full of sexual desire and that at any moment I'd explode. Jack told me that he gets really turned on when he's driving for long stretches. The vibration of the seat makes his balls ache, and he always winds up thinking about sex. He laughed and called it "diesel dick."

I don't know why we didn't just jump each other right away. He had no idea how turned on I was getting by just the idea of what I was doing. He couldn't have known. We probably spent ten or fifteen minutes just chatting and watching the movie, as if we were on a date or interested in the plot.

It was fairly explicit porn, not really my style. Lots of girl-on-girl stuff and hard, fast fucking. I guess that's what guys want—right to the point and the dirtier the better—but I've always been turned on by the idea of sex just as much as by the physical act. The mental aspect has always excited me, especially if I'm doing it somehow or somewhere I shouldn't be. Maybe that's why I was invited to do this dare.

I knew Jack was ready because his breathing was changing and he was spending more time staring intently at the TV. At first he had just glanced at it, kind of embarrassed to keep his eyes on it. But now, like me, he was getting so turned on that his desire was taking over. He was lying behind me on his side, spooning me, when he finally began to touch me in a sexual way. His hands slid down my arm before moving to my chest. I remember letting out a sigh and just lying back as he explored me, offering my breasts to him, just giving in to whatever he wanted and however he wanted it. God, it was so powerful. I don't remember ever wanting—needing—sex so badly, and here I was, pretending to be some indifferent hooker who's seen it all, done it all.

Then he asked me how much. The question caught me off guard, and I had to remind myself what I was pretending to be. I asked him exactly what he wanted to do, and he said, "I want it all." I had no idea what to say or what to charge. I told him I thought he was hot, so I'd give him a discount: a hundred dollars. He grinned. I didn't know if I was charging too much or too little, so I just grinned back in the same way. He reached into his wallet, which was tucked into the side of the mattress, and took out some twenties. He put them on the dash beside the pager.

Then, in a flash, all the pretense was gone. He began to rub my breasts, squeezing them in his hands and moving them around, then quickly sat up and peeled off his T-shirt. His body looked so good to me. I stayed on my back as he pulled my shirt off over my head, then reached under my back to unfasten my bra and expose my breasts. It felt wonderful.

I was just reveling in the exposure when his mouth came down on one of my nipples. He started biting at it, and it hurt just enough to make the pleasure build fast and strong. I looked down when his lips came off my nipple and saw how long and hard it was. I felt so filthy, just like a prostitute, but I'd never felt better. In that moment I learned something about myself. I learned that I'd have done anything that guy wanted just to fuck his body.

His body was so unfamiliar that his heavy breathing in my ear made my hips gyrate involuntarily. It made it better that he was a stranger. Everything was new and unexpected. I didn't know how he'd kiss, what his cock would look like, or how he'd fuck, but I couldn't wait to find out. While he was sucking hard on my nipple, I pushed my hips up toward him and pressed against his hardness. The feel of that wonderful bulge so close to my pussy drenched me instantly, and I told him so.

He liked hearing me talk like that, and he sat up quickly, snaking out of his jeans and shorts as fast as he could. I sat up and panted, staring at his cock and licking my lips. It was huge, thick and long and erect, and more than I ever could have hoped for. I've never really bought into the "big is better" thing, but in the heat of it all, I wanted to see for myself if it was true.

He pushed me onto my back and lifted up the short skirt I was wearing, pulling down my panties with a force and desperation that made me squirm. He was moving fast, which normally might have scared me, but I wanted him to take me and use me to get himself off. He crouched between my legs, then grabbed my knees and spread them open. My pussy— pink, wet, and swollen—was totally open to him. The air hit it, and I could feel his eyes moving all over its petals. In an instant, I felt his mouth sucking and licking and biting at it.

I grabbed the sheets and dug the back of my head into the mattress, trying not to come on his face. No guy has ever done that to me so eagerly before. . . . I could feel his strong tongue circle my clit and slip into my pussy, darting in and out a few times. Then he took it out and sucked my clit the same way he had sucked my tits, until it was thick and long, and again I thought I would burst.

He sat up for moment to touch my breasts, and I caught another glimpse of his beautiful cock. The head was swollen, and I imagined how good it would feel when it finally split me open and sank into my body. He went back down, and when his tongue slipped into my pussy I lifted my hips to meet it. I let him tongue-fuck me for a while, then groaned for him to ease off because I didn't want to come yet.

He stopped and leaned back, then grabbed my hair and pulled my head toward his cock. I took as much of it as I could into my mouth and sucked like never before. He kept saying "Oh yeah, oh yeah," and thrusting into my mouth, pumping his slick shaft between my tight lips. He wanted it so bad that his desire was turning me on even more. He started talking really dirty, saying things like "I'm fucking your mouth" and "I'm going to come down your throat," and his words made me frantic.

I gave him the best blow job any man could ask for, and I absolutely loved doing it. I sucked hard, pulling his cock out of my mouth with a loud pop, *then swallowed as much of the hard flesh as I could, sliding my lips down the slippery shaft and lapping the thick tip with my tongue. He tasted delicious, and I couldn't get enough of him. His sac was swollen and ready to explode. I squeezed his balls and tugged at the sac as I sucked his cock, and I felt his whole body shake above me in response.*

I was going to let him come in my mouth, but he suddenly pushed my head away and positioned me on my hands and knees. He said he wanted to have me from behind. I pulled my skirt up and he rubbed my ass with his hand, feeling me out. He pushed his hand between my legs and sank two fingers deep inside me. I shuddered and gasped at the feeling of sudden penetration, and I felt my wetness run down my thighs. Then with one fast thrust, he pushed his whole, huge cock inside. I wasn't expecting it, and I fell forward onto the mattress. With his cock still inside, he grabbed my hips and pulled me back up onto my knees. He was so big that I could feel his hardness fill every inch of my pussy, stretching and stimulating it like never before.

He started pumping so fast that it was all I could do to steady myself and stay on my knees, the sound of his grunts loud in my ears. He was very strong, and he was so turned on that he either didn't know or didn't care how hard he was doing it to me. He reached up and grabbed both of my shoulders, using them as leverage to drive himself deeper and harder inside me. It was so filthy, fucking like that, like animals. I wanted it to last forever. I was getting sore from how hard he was hitting me, and my breasts shook with each of his thrusts. All I could hear were my own moans, his grunts, and the slapping of our bodies coming together. I knew neither one of us would last much longer.

He let out a low, long groan, and his rapid thrusts changed to slow and deliberate as he erupted inside me. I could feel waves of come jet out of his cock and fill me up. It was warm and wet, and as soon as I felt it slide over my clit, I had an intense orgasm that seemed to cripple my body with pleasure. It lingered for a long time, and he kept sliding in and out of me, milking himself to the last drop and letting me enjoy him to the very end.

We lay down beside each other and caught our breath. Jack told me how good I had felt, and then got a couple of beers from a small fridge he had back there. I don't think a drink has ever tasted that good, and we just lay back and drank, with the porn still playing on the TV. I told him I had to go, then grabbed the cash and the pager and got out of the truck. The sun was just starting to come up.

The limousine was waiting for me just a few yards away, and I collapsed into the backseat. The chauffeur congratulated me, then asked me to write out my experience in detail. He said that I was now an initiate and that my dare would be shared with the rest of the group. He also said that now I'd get to read other initiates' stories. I can't wait for that.

Right now, I feel like I'm waking from a dream or a trance and I have so many questions. I still know very little about this organization that I am now a part of, and I certainly don't know how I had the courage to do what I did. I have no idea what to expect now or what's expected of me, but I'm up for another challenge, anytime, anywhere.

Thank you for this incredible experience. I truly hope you enjoyed reading my initiation dare, because I loved doing it.

The Music Store

Male, thirty-one

NEW YORK, NEW YORK

The chauffeur parked in front of a large music store and turned around in his seat to hand me two CDs. My instructions were to go to the back of the store, where the listening stations were, and to stand beside a woman listening with a headset. The chauffeur told me to put one of his CDs into the player and listen to it, and then to remove whatever disc the woman was listening to and put the other CD into her player.

I asked the chauffeur what was on the CDs, and he said it was sounds of people having sex. When the sex CDs were in both players, I was to initiate mutual masturbation with the woman, right there at the listening stations.

The consequences came flooding into my head, and I was really close to backing out. It was way too risky. What if the woman screamed or called the police? The chauffeur took one of the CDs out of my hand and put it into the limo's CD player. The sounds of sex—groans, moans, grunts, and sighs— swelled inside the car. My flesh tingled, and I felt a stir of arousal between my legs. I thought how good hands would feel on my groin, and I felt braver.

The promise of sex can make you do anything. The chauffeur ejected the CD and handed it back to me. I took it and got out of the limo. It was warm outside, so I took off my jacket and stared at the storefront. I felt more alive than I had in years and more virile than ever. It would be worth the risk.

My balls were tight as I entered the store, and walking was uncomfortable. The listening stations were at the back, just like the driver had described: six stations with stools and headsets. The store was moderately busy, and I wandered the aisles until a woman went to the listening stations and put on a headset. She had short blond hair and was attractive enough. She was lost in her music, oblivious as I came and stood right beside her and put my CD in. The sound hit me. The sound of a woman gasping in my ear, climaxing. My cock twitched.

I lifted one of the earphones off and leaned toward the woman to catch her attention. She smiled and took her headset off. "Try this," I said in a friendly voice, as I inserted the second CD into her player. "It's what I'm listening to, and it's great."

"Sure, thanks," she said and started to listen.

I held my breath, waiting for but fearing her reaction. She drew in a sharp breath. I stood frozen, waiting to see if she would run or call security, but she didn't move, and in that second I knew I had her. I knew it. My cock got hard, and my erection strained against my pants. She kept listening.

I fixed my eyes on her, and she glanced back, sizing me up and weighing the situation. I looked down at the bulge in my pants, and she followed my gaze. Then the incredible happened: She grinned. It was barely noticeable, but it was dangerous, and I knew she was game. Just like that.

That was the single most incredible moment of my life, the most incredible realization I've ever had: that I could walk up to a complete stranger and appeal to that part of her and that I could win her. It was a rush of excitement, power, and pleasure.

I looked up for security cameras and saw two pointing in

the opposite direction. "It'll never be risk free," I told myself. "It'll never be completely safe." That was the point. That was the dare. I ran my hand down my thigh and then back up to my groin. The woman watched as I touched myself, rubbing my bulge and toying with my zipper.

I saw her bite her bottom lip as I finally unzipped my pants and slipped my fingers inside. The feel of my fingers against my throbbing cock was electric, and the thrill of publicly exposing myself to a stranger made the sensation even stronger. The head of my cock pushed through, and the cool air of the room hit it. The woman stared at it but still didn't move.

I forced myself to reach out and touch the zipper of her jeans. I expected her to react in some way, either to resist or to help, but she did neither. She just stood there and stared at me, her expression totally blank. With both hands, I unbuttoned her jeans and unzipped them. She didn't stop me. She was wearing white cotton panties, and a lightning bolt of pleasure struck my cock when I saw them.

The heavy breathing and moaning in my ears and in hers was irresistible. I don't think anyone could've listened to it and left without release. I could hear the slapping of bodies coming together, the thrusts of a man penetrating a woman, the uncontrolled groans of ecstasy, and the wet sounds of sucking. It was too much.

Driven on by the sounds, I shoved my fingers down the front of her jeans and pressed them against her pussy. I could feel the moisture of her juices soaking through her panties. I felt her clit through the fabric and massaged it with my fingertip. Past the point of turning back or caring if I got caught, I twisted my wrist and moved the crotch of her panties aside to sink two fingers deep into her pussy.

The woman couldn't keep up her stone face anymore, and she rocked her hips toward me. She lowered her body to push my fingers deeper into her, and then reached out and squeezed my cock. My God, it was all I could do to not burst come into her palm right then. The pleasure bordered on pain. The filthy sounds and the risk of getting caught made it the most powerful sexual encounter anyone could ever experience.

The woman spooned my hand with her own until her fingers were juicy. Then she grabbed my cock and made my shaft slick with her juices. She dipped herself a few more times so her hand stroked smoothly, while all the while, I teased her. I tapped her clit, fingered the wet lips of her pussy, then pushed my fingers up into her.

She then started the most paralyzing rhythm I've ever felt. Her left hand squeezed the base of my cock hard enough to hurt, before she pulled up with a pinch on the head. Barely letting me penetrate her closed fist, she again went down my shaft. Then again. And again. Again.

It took less than a dozen of her strokes to make it build. Only a few more, and I erupted. The come rocketed out of my cock like never before. It racked my body, making me arch my back and almost groan out loud. I knew she was coming, too. She gyrated her body down onto my fingers, moving her hips in circles and breathing heavily. She kept stroking me the whole time, squeezing out every drop. I felt the extra moisture run down my fingers, and I knew she was finished.

She did her pants up and left quickly without looking back. I thought about taking the CDs, but the security cameras were turning and I didn't want to look suspicious, so I didn't. I left the store, and the chauffeur congratulated me, al-

though I don't know how he knew I'd actually completed the dare. He told me to write down what happened in the store, and that somebody from the group would be in contact soon.

The whole thing only took five or six minutes. Yet without a doubt, those were the most incredible, potent minutes of my life. I'm so glad I went through with it. I look forward to hearing from the group and to what comes next.

The Train

Male, forty, and Female, thirty-seven
DENVER, COLORADO

My wife and I were out for dinner when the waiter approached us at about ten P.M., and told us that a limousine was waiting for us outside. We couldn't believe the time had really come. We drove around in the limo for a while, until the chauffeur suddenly pulled over next to a train station. He said, "Your instructions are to get on the train, find a woman sitting alone, and proposition her for a threesome." He said there were a number of motels in the area we could use.

I could tell by the way my wife was laughing and moving her body that she was excited by the idea. I definitely was. We got out of the limo and took the next train. There were several women on it, but none turned my wife on. Even looking around like that was amazing, and my dick started to pound hard in anticipation.

We sat at the back of the train and talked about how we were going to approach somebody. How do you ask somebody that? "Hey, how'd you like to get a room and have sex with us?" Or

"Hey, my wife thinks you're hot, and it's my birthday. . . ." We didn't have a clue to what we'd say when the right woman came along.

After a few stops, a woman in a short skirt got on the train and sat down ahead of us. I knew by the way my wife watched her that she could be our girl. We decided that it might be better if my wife went up to her, so I sat back and watched as she moved to the seat next to the woman. It made me so hard watching my own wife do that, just knowing that she was trying to find me another woman to fuck. My wife tried to strike up a conversation, but the girl didn't seem to be into it, so she gave up pretty fast. The girl got off at the next stop.

We were determined to try again. It made us brave to do it that first time. After all, even though the lady didn't go for it, nobody had noticed anything and everything was safe. At the next stop, a woman in a business suit got on and sat across from us. It was perfect. She was perfect. My wife struck up a friendly conversation, and soon we were all chatting. The woman asked where we were heading, and my wife said, "We're just looking for a little harmless fun, but we need another player for what we have in mind . . . Do you have any plans?"

It took a second to register, but then the lady got it. She kept blinking and smoothing down the front of her pants. My wife said, "If you're not in a hurry, why not get a room with us, and we'll just see what happens?" The lady nodded, and I started visualizing myself pounding her with my wife on the bed right beside us. We jumped off at the next stop and checked into the first scummy motel we came across.

The three of us climbed a rickety flight of stairs until we arrived at room number seven. "Lucky number seven," I said, *and my wife chuckled and put her hand on the lady's back. We opened the door to the room, and that broke the ice: All of us laughed, since the room was exactly like the ones you see in the movies. It was small and dirty, with an old bed—no box spring—and a decrepit black-and-white TV in the corner.*

Yet there was something about the room that was turning all of us on. Strangers together in a seedy room for only one reason. The room was dirty, but so was our intention, and we were all getting more turned on by the second. At least I know I was. What guy hasn't dreamed about doing it with two women? We all exchanged glances, nervous at first, but soon we were more aroused than anxious. We couldn't wait to begin, but nobody was sure how to start or what we'd actually do. Sex is a natural thing, but it's awkward to get something like that started.

My wife took the lead and unbuttoned her blouse, then reached out and started to undress the lady. The lady didn't resist, and her head fell back on her shoulders, so we knew she was getting off on it. Soon they were both undressed, and I was standing there looking at two naked women. My wife has a curvy body with a small patch of dark pubic hair, but this woman had small breasts with a triangle of blonde hair between her legs, and I liked that they were so different. It felt so wrong to be looking at them, and that turned me on even more.

My wife threw herself on the bed and opened her legs, winking at me. I took my clothes off and held on to my dick, which was standing out from my body like a flagpole by that point, waiting for what came next. The whole thing was mind-blowing to watch. My wife spread her legs, and the lady started to eat her out. My wife was squirming and moaning and grabbing the lady's head, pushing her mouth onto her pussy. I stood looking right overtop and got a close-up of her getting tongued. Her clit was more swollen than I've ever seen it, and the lady kept sucking on it, making her groan really loudly. My wife was rubbing and pinching her own tits, a sight that made me lose control.

I climbed on top of my wife in the sixty-nine position and told her to suck me while I watched the other woman eat her out. I even pushed my fingers into my wife's pussy while the lady tongued it at the same time. We did that for a while, all of us poking and sucking, with my wife's hot mouth around my cock like never before. Each time I slid my finger into my wife, she'd suck even harder. I was surprised when she let out a scream and came hard, but I couldn't blame her for coming so fast.

My wife pushed me off of her and told me to fuck the other woman. I'd been aching to hear her say that. I pulled the lady onto her knees and started pounding her from behind as hard as I could, not really because I wanted to go that hard on her, but because I couldn't stop myself. It felt so different sinking my dick into another woman. The sight of her bare ass right in front of me, with my dick going in and out, was too much to bear.

I came close to coming a few times, and had to force myself to slow down, but that tight pussy hugging and squeezing my dick felt so good, and my wife kept urging me to go harder. I plunged into her again and again, and each time I got closer to orgasm. The woman was getting closer, too. I could tell by the way she pushed her ass back into me. My wife reached under me and squeezed my balls while I pumped the other woman's pussy.

You could almost taste the sex going on in that room. I was breathing hard and doing that woman harder than I've ever done it before. She let out a yell as she orgasmed and her pussy contracted around my cock. Between that feeling and my wife squeezing my balls, I couldn't stop from coming. I released my load into her body. It felt like hot lava shooting out of me, better and stronger than I could ever have imagined.

My wife and I collapsed onto the bed, but the woman only gathered her clothes and almost ran out of the room. We tried to tell her to stay and rest for a moment, but she took off. I don't know if she was embarrassed or if she just got what she came for and there was no reason to stick around. We dozed awhile but were woken up by a knock at the door. It was the chauffeur. He asked us to recount the details of our threesome, and that is what we have done.

Hopefully whoever reads this will get some pleasure out of it. We definitely don't have any regrets for accepting this dare, even though we've never done anything like this before. We'd be happy to do another one, as long as we're together.

Lube Job #17

◉

The Checklist—Sexual Positions

If you've ever taken your vehicle to a drive-thru lube station, you were probably handed your car's checklist when the job was done: it's the itemized list of services, from the hot-oil change to the brake fluid top-up, the techs performed on the engine. This checklist not only informs you of what's been done, it also reminds the tech of what he or she has to do. Personally, I don't seem to ever leave the house without a list in my pocket: buy a birthday present for my nephew, pick up Don's contacts at the optometrist's office, return my son's library books, drop off our taxes at the accountant's, find those drops that are supposed to heal the fish's eye infection. No, it doesn't get any more exciting than that, not even for sex writers.

Modern life is lived in the fast lane, and almost all of us rely on lists of some sort, from the weekly grocery list to the everyday "to do" list; however, some of us have longer lists than others. Lydia, forty-five, a wife, working mother, and stepmom, had a list that would make most of us drop to our knees in exhaustion rather than admiration. But it wasn't just one list, for Lydia had perfected her own complex system of independent and interrelated lists that covered every aspect of her home, family, work, and recreational life. This accomplishment had earned her the title of Lydia the List Lady, and it was by this name that her friends and family often referred to her.

To the dismay of her husband, Neil, forty-four, and the five teenage children under their roof, Lydia's list rampage had a long reach. Every morning, she would hand each member of the family his or her own list of things to do, clean, buy, fix, finish, and so forth. Every night, she would collect all the lists and amend them based on what was actually accomplished or on what new items needed to be added. In the morning, the lists were redistributed to their rightful holders. Sound effective? Probably, to some extent. Sound fun?

Lydia and Neil had been married for eight years. It was the second marriage for both of them, and they shared their home with the children from their first marriages: Lydia's three daughters were thirteen, fifteen, and eighteen, while Neil's daughter and son were thirteen and sixteen, respectively. Both Lydia and Neil expressed great satisfaction with their marriage as well as with the blended-family situation.

"Lydia would do anything for my kids, and I would for hers, too," says Neil. "Neither one of us did a very good job picking our first spouses, but we both wised up with our second. I can't complain about how Lydia treats my kids. Even when she's going crazy with her lists, she doesn't bark orders or act like a dictator. I think she's just overwhelmed since she's started back to work full-time, and she's desperate to find a way to get all the little things done. Everyone adores Lydia and tries to stick to his or her list, but she does go overboard sometimes."

"I like things to be in order," says Lydia, "I like the house to be clean; I like the fridge to be full of healthy food; I like the kids to be on time for all their different sports and activities. When you have a house full of five teenagers you're *always always always* hopping. Your life is in the details. You have to maximize every second, and you have to prioritize, which is why I keep lists for everything. It's the only way to make sure everything gets taken care of. As soon as you start slacking off, things get missed."

Like sex, for example.

"Neil's been known to add 'sex' to my list when I'm not looking," says Lydia. "I'd usually laugh and ignore it. I used to think he was just joking and that he was doing it just to get a laugh more than anything. I never really stopped to think about the fact that he wasn't getting much sex, and I'd say I definitely underestimated how important it was to him. I wasn't missing it, so it wasn't on my list. That meant it wasn't on his list, either."

"Of course I missed it," says Neil, "and there were times I'd feel bent out of shape about not getting it as often as I wanted. I'd jot 'sex' down on her list and cross my fingers she'd get the point, but she just shrugged it off. Then she'd be off doing something for one of my kids, so I'd feel like an ass for getting mad at her."

Somehow, Lydia's listmania didn't alienate her from her children or stepchildren, although she wonders how that was possible. "Those kids had a lot of tolerance for their ages," she says. "I'd push a list into their hands every single morning, and they'd just grit their teeth and say, 'Thanks.'"

In fact, it was Lydia's kids and stepkids who inadvertently led her to examine her own list of priorities.

"It was Mother's Day, and we were all sitting at the dining-room table having dessert. I was opening presents, and when I opened one of the cards, a really long list fell out. The kids had all gotten together and made a list of the things they loved about me, and how much they appreciated me. I couldn't hold back the tears. It was probably the most beautiful gift I've ever been given, and I remember exactly how it felt to be noticed like that."

> ✻ Thanks to the efforts of a woman named Anna Jarvis, President Woodrow Wilson declared Mother's Day a holiday in 1914. But Anna Jarvis soon became outraged by the commercialism of the holiday and was arrested for disturbing the peace at a convention where white carnations—her own mother's favorite flower—were being sold for profit.

The list did more than make Lydia cry; it also made her realize how far out of order her priorities really were. "I had such a feeling of validation and importance when I read that list. I wanted Neil to have that same feeling of importance, but when I started to think about it, I realized that I wasn't treating him as a priority. I read the two lists I was working on for him. One was called House, and the other was Yard. Spring break was coming up, and since all the kids would be gone to their other parents' houses, I was planning to get a lot done around our house. The lists included things like buy new garden hose, check sump pump, paint the downstairs baseboards. It suddenly seemed insane. We had five days together *without the kids,* and I was thinking about the sump pump?"

So Lydia the List Lady started two new lists for Neil. The first was called Love, and the second was called Sex. The Love list contained all the things Lydia would concentrate on to show her husband that he was a priority in her life. The list read as follows:

The Love List

- ♥ Kiss you and tell you I missed you when you get home
- ♥ Thank you for working so hard and being a great husband and dad
- ♥ Focus on giving you more love and fewer lists
- ♥ Let you have time away with your friends whenever possible
- ♥ Be less critical
- ♥ Relax and let you relax
- ♥ Get my priorities straight
- ♥ Make time for date nights (without the kids!)
- ♥ Ask what you'd like to do, instead of always telling you what to do
- ♥ Remind myself often how much and why I love you

- ♥ Learn more about your goals for the future
- ♥ Save some time and energy at the end of the day just for you
- ♥ Always treat you with respect in front of the kids
- ♥ Look my best for you
- ♥ Treat you as a person, not just my husband

"I wanted to remind Neil and myself that we were in love," says Lydia. "It's scary how you can almost forget that, even if you're happy. You have to remember that you're lovers and partners as well as parents. Our kids are going to be gone in just a few short years, and I don't want us to be one of those couples who stare at each other across the table, thinking 'Now what do we do? Now what do we talk about? Who the hell are you, anyway?' A couple has to focus on staying in love in the midst of all the distracting details of life."

The Sex list was less sentimental, but just as moving.

"The Love list was all about emotion," explains Lydia, "but I knew Neil was feeling forgotten in a physical way, too. He was a man in need of some serious maintenance sex. I remembered all those times he'd scribbled 'sex' onto my lists, so I decided to give him what he wanted in a big way. I wanted him to be turned on just by reading it, so I made it a list he'd want to get to work on right away."

To that end, the Sex list contained a list of sexual positions that Lydia and Neil used to practice or had yet to try. Being a creative woman, Lydia even crowned some positions with their own unique titles. And although it's anyone's guess how some of these names looked in action, the list read as follows:

The Sex List

♂ The Battering Ram
♂ Rear Entry
♂ Leaning Tower of Pisa
♂ Sideways Slammer
♂ Doggy Style
♂ Standing
♂ Sitting
♂ The Scissors
♂ The Rocking Horse
♂ Bucking Bronco

"The Love list meant a lot to me," says Neil, "but I must admit it didn't get my attention like her Sex list did. I already knew Lydia loved me, but I was beginning to think that she wasn't that interested in sex with me anymore. It wasn't merely a turn-on to read the Sex list, it was also a huge relief. It was proof that she hadn't abandoned me sexually. And I couldn't wait to find out how some of those moves worked."

According to Neil, many women don't truly appreciate the fundamental connection between love and sex that exists for men. "Lots of guys can go out and have strictly sexual affairs and love isn't part of that, but in a marriage or a long-term monogamous relationship, sex and love go hand in hand. Once the sex starts to disappear, feelings of intimacy and love also start to go away. When Lydia and I would go two or three weeks without sex, I'd feel our connection stretching thin. Sex is kind of the glue that holds a man to a woman and makes the relationship stick together.

We're not being pigs; it's just how we are. When Lydia is sexual with me, I feel much more loved. And I almost hate to say it, but I'm more aware of my love for her."

"That's a big difference between men and women," says Lydia. "For me, the love list is far more meaningful than the sex list, but I realize that isn't necessarily so for men. Keeping them satisfied in the sex department instead of just saying how we feel shows them how much we love them. Maybe it's as simple as actions speak louder than words for men. That's why I now think maintenance sex is a lot more important than I used to. It never used to be on my list at all, but now it's always at the top. What do I care if the garden hose has a hole in it when my husband isn't feeling loved or satisfied? It's a matter of getting your priorities straight."

Well, if a hard-core list maker like Lydia can reconsider her priorities, so can the rest of us. Her checklist approach is a wonderful way for a woman to show her man that he is the most important part of her life and to give him a strong sense of worth. Why not make your own Love list, tailored to suit your life together, and give it to your partner? If you're always on the go, tell him you'll try to slow down and be more affectionate. If he never has any time to himself, tell him you'll try to give him more time to unwind, whether it's playing video games or shooting pool with his friends. Make sure your list lets him know how appreciated, needed, and respected he is as a man, not just as your partner.

Just when he thinks things can't get any better, give him a second list—a list of sexual positions—and tell him you can't wait to start checking off the positions with him!

Even if your relationship is a happy one, your man may on occasion feel more physically forgotten than you realize. A Sex list is an erotically effective way to show him that you've remembered his needs and that you're committed to fulfilling them. It's also a wonderful way to emotionally and sexually validate your man and to bulletproof your relationship.

This lube job describes a number of sexual positions you may wish to include in your Sex list, but don't be afraid to jot down a few zigzags you'd like to test drive. The excitement of a new or unusual sexual position is an easy way to add a sexy twist to lovemaking. Men find it very arousing to see and feel a woman's body move in different ways and especially to experience penetration at different angles.

> **Clear the clutter off the dresser so your man can watch in the mirror as he penetrates you in different positions. To make your bedroom an erotic fun house, position a number of mirrors around the bed so he can get a 360-degree view of all the action. He'll be the star of his own show.**

To use your Sex list for maintenance purposes, place it in your man's keeping and tell him to present it to you when he's in need. If you're energetic, you can complete the list in one sweaty sex session. Or the two of you can work down the list over time, checking off each position as you go. When you give your man the list, you provide him with a straightforward yet guiltless way to express his needs and ask for sex. That's a bigger gift than you might think.

The positions described below are fairly tame (sorry, no swinging from the chandeliers or Olympic-gymnast backflips); however, they should be enough to please or at least to inspire you to explore a few new angles on your own. Of course, only you can judge your physical abilities, and if there are moves you don't feel comfortable trying, skip them or adapt them to suit your abilities and preferences.

Consider some of the following moves in your sex list. If you're feeling creative, you can give each one your own personalized title, as Lydia did.

1. From behind: Man lying on top of woman.

Lie facedown on the bed, and have your partner lie on top of you. To help him penetrate you, place a pillow under your body to lift your bum off the bed. This will also make your vagina feel tighter as he enters you. Your man can thrust while lying flat on top of you, or he can sit up and straddle your body while you lie facedown. When he sits up, ask him to grab your hips or squeeze your buttocks as he thrusts into you; you'll both love it. And since this position is a great one for stimulating the G-spot, you won't be bucking him off.

2. Woman on top: Man lying on back, woman straddling him.

Men love this one, since they get to lie back while you do all the work. Have your man lie on his back, then straddle his erect penis and lower yourself onto it, guiding it into your body with your hand. If you're tall, it might be sufficient for you to lift and lower yourself while on your knees; however, if you're petite, you may have to squat and use leg power to raise and lower yourself. Make a spectacle of pumping your man in this position, since the more enthusiastic you are—the more you bounce and grind—the more turned on he'll be. Let him really get off on the sight of your naked breasts and body towering above him: play with your nipples, arch your back to really get those breasts out there, and slide a finger down to enjoy the feel of his penis entering you.

To add some sexy variety, lean back until your body is resting on outstretched arms. Move your feet up closer to your partner's head for stability, then use your arms and legs to rock up and down, pumping your man's penis. This lean-back position changes the angle of penetration and varies sensation.

3. Woman lying on back, man kneeling.

Lie on your back and raise your legs straight in the air, with your feet resting on your man's shoulders. To help entry and make your vagina feel tighter, place a thick pillow under your bum. If you prefer, keep your legs closed and rest both your feet on one of your partner's shoulders instead. He can wrap his arms around your legs to steady your body as he thrusts into you. He can even lift up your legs (whether they're closed or open) to raise your body higher and play even more with the angle of penetration.

To detour into an easy variation, open your legs so your man can lean forward over your body to rest on his outstretched arms. This will bring your legs up over your head, which will in turn facilitate some delicious deep penetration.

After a while, you may wish to return to your original close-legged position. Have your man kneel back up, then bend your knees and tuck them in close to your chest. Your partner can use your kneecaps for support as he thrusts into you. Be sure to keep your knees bent and your legs tightly together. Slight changes like this are easy and, if made midstride, will affect the way penetration feels for both of you and keep your excitement level up.

4. Standing: Woman's back against the wall.

If you're able to pull it off, this one's nasty. (In the best way, of course.) Wrap your legs around your man and either hold on to his shoulders tightly or wrap your arms around his neck to stop your body from sliding down his. Your back should be straight against the wall, and if he presses your body against the wall hard enough while he thrusts, that will also help you from slipping. Tell him to lift you by your buttocks as he thrusts. Don't worry if you can't sustain this position for too long or until orgasm; you can always transfer the festivities to the floor and finish in another position.

5. Missionary.

The missionary position—with the woman lying on her back and the man lying on top of her, face-to-face—has an undeservedly bad reputation, not unlike maintenance sex itself. As long as you don't lie there like a cold dead fish, the missionary position has great erotic potential. You can look into your man's eyes to show him your enraptured expression; you can kiss his mouth, neck, face and shoulders; and you can run your hands all over his back, shoulders, and even his chest when he lifts his body up a bit. So don't slander this position unnecessarily. Wrap your legs around your man's body, run your nails down his back, kiss his throat, and whisper sweet nothings (or dirty thoughts) into his ear as he thrusts.

For an easy on-the-fly change, alternate between opening your legs wide and squeezing them tightly closed as he penetrates you from above. Or, keep your legs together and twist your body until you're more or less lying on your side.

6. Doggy style.

Ah, don't you just love the classics? Of course, in this time-tested favorite, you're on all fours as your man kneels behind you and penetrates you from behind. He can grab onto your shoulders or hips for leverage if he wants to go harder or faster. To add to your pleasure, have your man reach around to stimulate your clitoris while he thrusts. To increase his excitement, as he thrusts push your bum back against him to show him just how good he feels inside you.

Or reach underneath to squeeze his testicles or fondle his perineum. You can also ask him to lift one of your legs and hold on to it by the thigh as he thrusts. This will let him go deeper and will make your clitoris easier to reach for stimulation.

7. Sitting: Man and woman face-to-face.

Like the missionary position, this one lets you and your man enjoy intercourse while facing each other. Have your man sit upright on the bed (or on the edge of the bed with his legs hanging over the side) and swing one of your legs over his lap so that you're sitting on top of him, face-to-face. Use your hand to guide his penis inside you. Either hold on to his shoulders or wrap your arms around his neck to help lift your body up off his penis and then lower it back down. You'll have to do most of the work, but this is such a sweetly intimate position that you won't mind. Take advantage of this face-to-face time by kissing your man deeply on his mouth, neck, and shoulders. Gyrate your hips to add extra sensation.

8. Front to back: Man lying on back, woman lying on top of him, on her back.

This is another one the boys really love. Have your man lie flat on his back, then lie flat on top of him, on your back, with your head over his. He can now reach up and around to feel your naked breasts and body on top of him. It may take some minor maneuvering to slip his penis inside, but it's worth the effort. Thrusting is best kept slow and sure in this exquisite position.

9. Woman on top: Woman straddling man, facing his feet.

Have your man lie flat on his back with his legs straight out, and then straddle his body, facing his feet. This position allows him to enjoy the sight of your naked back and bum on top of him and is a great spin on the standard woman-on-top. By facing his feet, you change the angle of penetration and the feel of his thrusts. To play with the angle still more, lean forward (toward his feet) and push yourself back onto his penis, pumping. As a variation, have your man spread his legs. Squat between them with your knees together and your hands on his knees, and use his knees as support to raise and lower yourself onto his penis.

10. The wheelbarrow: Woman standing on her hands, man standing on his feet.

This one isn't as difficult as it sounds—honestly! (Although it's more of a challenge if you're a lot shorter than your partner.) Get onto your hands and knees on the floor, and then have your man lift your legs up until he's holding you by your thighs. As you support yourself on your hands, he pulls your vagina onto his penis. While this might sound like a lot of effort, it really isn't, as long as you aren't too heavy. And sex doesn't always need to be a leisure activity. Don't be afraid to work up a sweat now and then.

As you work through this or your own list of sexual positions, don't become preoccupied with perfect form. The excitement comes from the novelty of the effort, not flawless positioning. If you can't bend that/hold that/lift that/do that, then try something else. If a move just doesn't do anything for you or your partner, slide into the next one.

If your down-filled pillows don't provide the sexual support you need, you might find an actual *sex pillow* more helpful. These specially designed, very supportive pillows are available in different shapes and sizes to facilitate new angles of penetration. Prop one under your chest or hips, kneel on it, or even straddle it with your partner. The possibilities are endless, and you'll love exploring them together.

The feel and sight of your bodies together in different ways—moving, touching, thrusting, watching—is what ramps arousal. So gear your man up for a night of sharp turns.

Lube Job #18

●

The Backseat Drive-In—Sex in the Car

Some of the most special times a couple shares are the result of a last-minute change in plans, a spur-of-the-moment decision, or an unplanned whirlwind vacation. Spontaneity is freedom. It reminds a couple that they have some control over their lives, that they aren't slaves to their routine, and that they exist as man and woman independently of their children or other responsibilities. When a couple takes an unplanned detour they sometimes find not only that the experience is fun, but also that it creates a lifelong memory that strengthens their history together.

Most of us have these kinds of memories: that wrong turn that brought us to the best cheeseburger joint we'd ever found; that movie we rented by accident that turned out to be hilarious; that garage sale we decided on a whim to stop at, only to find the rare stained-glass window that now adorns the front door to our home. Spontaneous sexual experiences can also be the most memorable. Remember the first time your man leaned in to kiss you or the night you shared a ravaging stand-up quickie against the refrigerator of your first apartment?

Sadly, sexual spontaneity fades from a long-term couple's life as the routine of work, home, kids, worries, chores, bills, whatever, takes over. Often, it disappears completely, and the loss is one to be grieved. Fortunately, we can resurrect this pale memory from our past and breathe new life into it. All it takes is a playful spirit and a willingness to throw the almighty routine into the backseat once in a while. And nowhere is this attitude more useful than in the performance of maintenance sex.

> **Is sex more annoying than arousing? It might just be bad timing that has you growling. Practice "planned spontaneity" by letting your man know the best and worst times to initiate sex with you. After date night = good. On the phone with Mom = bad. If he makes the moves when you're apt to be receptive, his odds will improve.**

Darren and Jenny were a busy working couple complete with two adult children, two child-substitute spaniels, matching laptops, and a frighteningly comprehensive knowledge of mutual funds who were admitted kiss-your-feet slaves to a brutal dictatorship routine of work and play. Sex, however, wasn't part of the regime.

"I was going through early menopause and just wasn't that interested in sex," admits Jenny, forty-six. "Combine that with a recent job promotion and an extra ten or fifteen hours a week at the lab, and I really couldn't have been less interested in lovemaking. Darren would bring it up at times, mostly asking if I needed hormone replacement to get back in the mood. It was my decision to go through menopause without medical intervention. Looking back, it was a somewhat selfish decision. I went months without wanting sex, and Darren's needs just fell off my radar screen."

So what brought the blip of Darren's sexual needs back onto the screen?

"I was in his e-mail account for an innocent reason when I noticed a subject line that read 'Fly away with me!' I opened it and found it was from a neighbor of ours. She was laughing about an occasion when they'd bumped into each other while dog walking. They'd taken the alley back to our street and stumbled across some kids trying to get a kite out of a tree. I guess Darren climbed up and got it down, and then they went back to the park and flew the kite with the kids for a while. It sounded like they'd had a lot of fun. I couldn't remember the last time Darren and I had that kind of experience, and I felt jealous I hadn't shared it with him. He hadn't mentioned any of it to me, and I must admit I felt insecure about it. I didn't even know she had his e-mail address."

Jenny had reason to be concerned; the woman her husband had bumped into was well known among the wives in the neighborhood for having had an affair with a married man. She was not the type of neighbor the ladies on the block had over for an afternoon coffee.

"Her reputation preceded her," says Jenny, "but I

shouldn't have been worried. The fact that I was worried sent my red flags up, and I took a good look at my marriage. I realized that I, and my marriage, had become boring, predictable, and celibate. Darren was a forced celibate."

> Many women experience a loss of sexual desire during menopause or perimenopause, primarily due to hormonal imbalances of estrogen, progesterone, and testosterone. Vaginal dryness, mood swings, and fatigue are also common, which can further lower the libido and put a strain on your sex life. Help is available, so see your doctor.

Jenny deleted the e-mail, added the naughty neighbor to the blocked sender's list, and didn't bring the issue up with Darren. Instead, she sprang into immediate action.

"Talk is cheap," says Jenny. "I'm all about results. Anyway, it wasn't conversation that we needed to engage in. I stopped Darren on the stairs. He was heading to the basement to work out, but I asked him to come with me instead. We got into the car and I drove straight to the adult video store. I parked outside, and he started laughing so hard I thought he was going to have a stroke on me. He was grinning like the cat who ate the canary. I told him to go in and pick something and to hurry; it was showtime."

Darren returned to the car carrying his bag of eye candy, and Jenny began to drive home. It was early evening, the sun was setting, and the couple was fully enjoying the sense of liberty their spontaneous trip to the XXX movie store had given them when an unexpected detour presented itself.

"Darren was laughing and reading the back of the DVD covers," recalls Jenny. "We were getting turned on and having a great time when he reached to the floor of the backseat and grabbed my laptop. I had forgotten it was in the car. He winked and took it out of its case, then inserted the DVD. He asked me when I last went to a drive-in movie. Before I knew it we were driving down the road with this porno playing."

Instead of telling him to turn it off and wait until they got home, Jenny quickly recognized the experience for what it was: an exciting opportunity for sexual spontaneity. Without giving herself enough time to reconsider, she pulled into the back parking lot of an out-of-business electronics store.

"We were in the middle of the city, but there was nobody around us," says Jenny. "We climbed into the backseat with the laptop and had our own private showing. I can't believe what I've been missing, but that was the first time I ever had intercourse in the car. I never even made out in a car when I was a teenager. Now, at forty-six, I'm doing it in the backseat of a luxury sedan with my husband and a porno. That's style! After twenty-some years of marriage, we're kids again, and we're loving it."

Jenny's story is a great one, but there's no reason you have to wait for your man's sexual needs to fall off your radar screen before you treat him to the X-rated drive-in theater experience. You don't need a luxury sedan or a laptop computer, either. Even the most utilitarian, unsexy, soccer ball–filled, cookie-smeared minivan equipped with that child-friendly portable DVD player in the backseat can play host to a sinful night of adult viewing and memory-making maintenance sex.

Once your in-car movie screen (whether a laptop or a DVD) is ready to light up the dashboard, ask your man to take a midnight drive. You might want to stash some lube and personal cleansing wipes in the glove box. After you find a safe, secluded spot, park, lock the doors, and press play.

> The first movie shown in a drive-in theater was called *Wife Beware*. It played in Camden, New Jersey, in 1933.

It's up to you whether you want to start things off in the front seat and then migrate to the back, or whether you want to camp out in the backseat from the beginning. If you start in the front, have your man push his seat all the way back, lean into his body, and kiss him deeply on the mouth, letting your hands explore his chest before moving down to his groin. Knead his inner thighs with your fingers and then rub his penis and testicles, maybe adding a gentle squeeze to get their full attention. Tell him how badly you want him as you unfasten his pants and expose his genitals. Take a handful of lube and apply it to his penis and testicles, rubbing it into his skin and pubic hair.

Sit back and undress yourself as your man watches by the romantic glow of the interior light. Swing your leg over his lap and straddle him. Lower yourself onto his penis just a little, just enough to feel him against your vagina. Circle your hips and press down as if you're going for penetration, then lift yourself back up, teasing him. Let him anticipate how good it will feel before you finally let him sink into you and start pumping. If you're slim enough, tell him to reach around you and hold on to the steering wheel for leverage as he thrusts up into you. You can also spin around so that you're holding on to the steering wheel while you pump him.

Climb off your man and clamber into the back of the car. Pull the rest of his clothes off and lie on your back on the backseat with your legs open and ready for him. As he lies on top of you and penetrates you, tell him to look at the screen. The sights and sounds of a dirty movie playing inside the car, combined with the intensity of this sexual experience, may bring him to the finish line faster than you expected.

While this drive may have started out as a pleasure trip designed for him only, its raw eroticism might have you asking your man to slow down and make the ride last longer. Such is the benefit of spontaneous maintenance sex. It's powerfully effective, and, before you know it, you might be the one who needs servicing. Either way, you've acquired a sexy memory that neither of you will soon forget. And the next time you pop a cartoon into that DVD player for the kids, you'll be able to share a saucy smile of remembrance with your man.

While we've suggested you choose an adult film as your drive-in movie, not all couples may wish to do so. If you're not comfortable with pornography, you can always choose a love story, perhaps one on the racier side, for a more sub-

> Can't find a babysitter? You don't have to leave home to go to this drive-in. Park the car in the garage, wait until the little darlings are asleep, and then slip into the garage for a quickie performance at your own theater. This is also a great alternative for those who, when it comes to sex, prefer private property to public parking.

tle approach. That being said, there are many couples who do enjoy pornography and who have managed to successfully integrate it into their sex lives.

If you're a porn virgin, why not consider dipping your toes into the adults-only waters just to see how they feel? Today's pornography industry offers viewers a great deal of choice in terms of content and style. You don't have to dive into hard-core orgies and unsavory close-ups. A warm wade into soft-core sex—perhaps a film by a female producer/director—may be a sexier and more female-friendly choice, especially for beginners. Many adult films are aimed at the couples' market, offering big-budget, high-quality movies with entertaining story lines and tasteful, egalitarian sex scenes.

Still, some women have concerns about using pornography in their intimate relationship. There's no doubt pornography, including the widespread practice of Internet sex surfing, has the *potential* to lead to a serious physical and emotional breakdown in a relationship, but it certainly doesn't always do so. As with anything, the best approach is moderation and communication.

We all know there are some men who take pornography (in any medium) to extremes and become obsessed with it, alienating their significant other in the process. Think of that guy who risks his job by downloading porn onto his work computer, or the man who destroys his personal life by spending hours downstairs on his home computer, printing volumes of XXX material instead of engaging with his wife and family. In those instances, the issue may have less to do with porn and more to do with personality or psychological problems. That's another book.

We'll limit our discussion here to the committed man who rents the occasional skin flick or sometimes views porn online (no chat rooms or cybersex, no underage, no violence) but who still engages in regular and mutually satisfying lovemaking with his woman. Basically, we're talking about the guy who might take the "free tour" before bed but who misses no opportunity to jump between the sheets with his woman. He sees porn as harmless, but she sees it as cheating. These polarized opinions usually stem from the differences between male and female sexuality. Communication is the path to finding that elusive middle ground where both people in the relationship are respected and understood.

Let's eavesdrop on a couple's "porn" talk:

WIFE: Why do you need to look at porn? Aren't I enough for you?

HUSBAND: Yes, you're enough. You're beautiful, but guys like to look at naked women. We're hardwired that way, it has nothing to do with you. It wouldn't matter who I was with, I'd still want to look every now and then.

WIFE: But if you look at those women, with their fake bodies and the best lighting, you'll expect me to look like that.

HUSBAND: I love the way you look. I'm more attracted to you than to any woman in the world, or I wouldn't be with you. I know what I see in porn isn't real. I know their breasts are implants; I know their skin is covered in makeup; and I know they don't really make those sounds when they're having sex. So no, I don't expect you to look like that. I don't even *want* you to look like that. In the same way, I hope you don't expect me to look like or last as long as the guys in porn films.

WIFE: Why do you sneak off to look?

HUSBAND: Because it's fun to look, but I don't want to hurt your feelings and I don't want you to think you're not good enough. I also feel that you'll judge me if I look at it.

WIFE: But if I let you watch it too much, you'll get addicted to it.

HUSBAND: Everything in moderation. It's no different than eating a chocolate bar. Most people will have one once in while but won't overeat until they're six hundred pounds. There are those guys who depend on porn to get off, but they're the extreme and most men aren't like that and don't want to be like that. Most of us just want to get our kicks now and then by looking at porn but think it's pathetic to be jerking off in front of the computer instead of making love to our own woman. You can't judge all men by a few insensitive and warped guys. It makes the rest of us look just as weird, when we're not, and that's not fair to us.

WIFE: What about what's fair to me? I feel unattractive, unloved, and inadequate when you look at porn.

HUSBAND: All I can do, as your loving partner, is put my arms around you and tell you how beautiful I think you are. But there are differences between men and women: we like to look, it really is that simple. It doesn't mean we want one of those girls or that we feel anything toward them. In fact, I could never pick one of the girls I'd seen in a porn out of a lineup. I watch it, get a thrill, then it's over. I'm not thinking about it anymore. Women think there's more to it than there is.

WIFE: Don't you think it's cheating to be looking at another woman's naked body?

HUSBAND: No, I don't. That's a matter of personal opinion, belief, and spirituality, but when I look at porn, I'm still devoted and faithful to you. If one of the stars were to jump out of the television and beg me to climb on top of her, I wouldn't do it.

WIFE: So what's the draw to porn?

HUSBAND: It's just the idea of watching other people have sex. It's kind of voyeuristic, and it turns me on. It's no different than the romance novels women read.

WIFE: There aren't any naked pictures of men in romance novels.

HUSBAND: No, but there's romance and hidden dirty scenes, because that's what turns women on. In porn, there's naked bodies and grunting, because that's what turns men on. Each medium appeals to its gender. Let me ask you something. After you're finished reading a romance novel, do you fall in love or become obsessed with the muscle-bound, poetry-reciting hero?

WIFE: Of course not.

HUSBAND: Do you compare me to him?

WIFE: No.

HUSBAND: Do you need to think about him to get turned on?

WIFE: No.

HUSBAND: It's the same thing. It's escapist.

WIFE: Do you want me to look at porn with you?

HUSBAND: I'd like to try it, just like we try other things like sex toys or different positions. There are lots of couple-oriented films and websites that we might find exciting to see together. Maybe then you'll understand that it's just a small part of my sexuality and that you're the woman who keeps me coming back for more. And if we watch it together, I can reassure you how much I love you.

Admittedly, this is an idealized conversation. That's okay, since it's intended to be as instructional as it is informative. Communication is the antidote for almost any ill in a relationship, and that includes the issue of pornography. If you and your partner are struggling with porn, you need to have an honest heart-to-heart, free of judgment and punishment. On one hand, you cannot expect to overrule your man's natural sexuality and dole out only the material you see fit without compromise. He's an individual, not just your partner, and that militaristic attitude may backfire. At the same time, your partner cannot be insensitive to or dismissive of your feelings as a woman. You need to know that you are loved, desired, adored, and preferred over any other woman in the world, and the material he views must not violate your values.

Now that you and your man have ascended to this lofty plane of higher communication, we can get back to the matter at hand, that is, maintenance sex and pornography. Remember that maintenance sex is as much about maintaining the strength of the relationship as it is about managing different sex drives. We're talking about *relationship* maintenance as opposed to just *man* maintenance. If you and your partner are both satisfied with a decision to go porn-free, you're set for sexual success. But if your man is craving a peek and you're covering his eyes, you may be in for problems.

Here's an idea—instead of allowing porn to divide you, why not see if it can bring you closer? In the next chapter, you'll see how sensual massage can be used to bridge the emotional, physical, and sexual distance between partners. By engaging in sensual massage while you watch an agreed-upon X-rated movie or surf a sexy site together, you'll be able to exploit the eroticism of the images but still maintain your intimate connection. It's a way to let your man indulge in this side of his sexuality without your feeling sidelined. If you can both agree on the rules (the type of material you view and how often you watch), you'll show your man that two-player porn is a better game than sexual solitaire. You might also find that you actually like playing along once in a while.

Introducing sensual touch into the porn experience may create an aura of intimate exploration where a woman who is uncertain about her partner's pro-porn activities can be comfortable joining in. And as for you porn veterans out there, why not watch the whole video for a change? Slow down, touch each other (not like that!), and delight in each other's bodies before you start playing monkey-see, monkey-do with the stars on the screen.

> The word *pornography* comes from the Greek word for prostitute. *The School of Whoredom*, a sixteenth-century pornographic novel, was written by Pietro Aretino, who is considered as the father of European pornographic writing. In this witty book, a mother who is an experienced courtesan teaches her daughter how to please a man.

Pornography can also serve as effortless foreplay to a no-frills maintenance quickie. We've all experienced those aroused versus exhausted nights when we want to relieve our partner's sexual pressure but don't have the energy to fully rev him up. On those occasions, a few minutes of pornographic viewing pleasure may be all that is required to get him ready for sexual release. Adding the lusty sights and sounds of an adult movie to even the most dutiful hand job can turn maintenance into magnificence. Choose an "emergency" adult film to buy with your partner and keep it handy for fast-and-easy maintenance sex purposes.

Whether you need to ease into the X-rated experience through sensual touch or you're ready to throw yourselves into the backseat of your car and watch a skin flick in an abandoned parking lot, well-chosen pornography has the potential to add an exciting and fulfilling dimension to your love life. Choose material you're comfortable with, view in moderation, and press play. Most important, be sure to use pornography in a fun and spontaneous way. It's a thrilling, adults-only way to happily maintain a long-term intimate relationship.

Lube Job #19

●

Fully Loaded—Sensual Massage

Like I am most mornings, I was running late. My son
was dawdling to hair-pulling extremes, and we had already missed the school bell. It had snowed the night before, and my car was frosted. Half a foot of snow was piled
on top of the roof, the windows were ice, and the driveway
was packed with heavy snow that was still falling. I
wrapped a scarf around my son's neck, grabbed his back-
pack, and raced to the car with my breath freezing as it hit
the cold air. The car's engine turned over—barely—and after I strapped my son into the backseat, I did a makeshift
job of scraping the ice and snow away before jumping behind the steering wheel and rubbing my hands together
for warmth.

I looked out the windshield. The car's defroster was
clearing the frost from the glass, but pounds of snow still
sat on the hood of the car, extending all the way up to the
windshield to cover the wipers. As I put my hand on the
wiper control to brush the snow away, I heard Don's voice

in my head: "Don't use the wipers if they're packed with snow, or you'll burn the motor out. Brush all the snow off before you turn them on. That motor's expensive to fix."

What does he know, I thought. I'm cold. I'm late.

I turned on the wipers, and the frozen motor groaned under the weight of the packed snow. For a moment, it looked promising: The wipers moved a quarter of an inch and I had visions of them sweeping upward, brushing the snow off the windshield to free me from my zero-visibility vehicular igloo. All would be well. The groaning grew louder for a moment, then silence. Not normal silence, mind you, but that special type of silence that accompanies an indefinable sense of defeat. The wiper motor was dead; the snow continued to fall.

And the motor was expensive to fix, after all. What's more, the wipers have never worked as well since the motor was replaced. Sometimes they come to our rescue in a downpour; sometimes they force us to pull over until the clouds pass. As some of us learn the hard way, a little preventative maintenance can avoid a lot of repairs later on, not to mention money, time, and frustration.

An ounce of prevention is worth a pound of cure. We hear this cliché so often that we fail to take it seriously, but nowhere is this truer than in our intimate relationships. Maintenance sex is about more than managing disparate sex drives; it's also about maintaining the relationship as a whole, and that's the focus of this chapter. For once a relationship has suffered a breakdown, particularly infidelity, it's a long and sometimes endless road to repair. Though the whys, whens, with whoms, and hows of infidelity are many, the following story is a good example of how sexual problems can factor into a stereotypical workplace affair.

In their midthirties and married for two years, Deanna and Marcus had spent more than half of their short marriage trying to have a child. Deanna had battled endometriosis in her twenties and was now fighting infertility in her thirties, and although she had managed to get pregnant twice, both pregnancies ended in early miscarriages. The loss and the continued disappointment of negative home-pregnancy tests took their toll on their relationship: love-making disappeared; baby making took over.

Happier skies seemed to be overhead when Deanna conceived a third time. The pregnancy, although burdened with around-the-clock morning sickness, was a strong one, and Deanna's obstetrician assured her their unborn daughter was fat and fabulous. Despite the baby's healthy progress, however, Deanna was preoccupied with her past miscarriages and sidelined by green-faced, unrelenting nausea, a combination that resulted in a very stressed mom-to-be. Sex became even more unimportant, at least to Deanna.

"For over a year, sex hadn't been about feeling good; it had been about conceiving," says Marcus. "Procreation, not recreation. She'd take her temperature, and if it was right, we'd do it. If not, we wouldn't. After she did get pregnant, sex wasn't as important to Deanna. As far as she was concerned, the goal was accomplished. For the first couple months of the pregnancy she wouldn't do it at all since she was afraid it would jeopardize the baby. I knew why she was so scared, but it was frustrating. There was no medical reason to abstain, but she still wouldn't have sex. I took it personally."

As the pregnancy progressed, and Deanna's nausea worsened, Marcus began to feel even more sexually unsatisfied. "I did my best to reassure her that the pregnancy was going to be all right. Her belly kept getting bigger, right on schedule, but she was still worried. I understood why, but as time went on, I got angry that the sex had stopped. I would've appreciated a hand job, and I would've bowed down at her feet for a blow job, but it wasn't happening. Sexually speaking, she was completely tuned out."

> **Spooning is a great position for intercourse during pregnancy. It keeps that growing belly out of the way, lets you stay intimate, and doesn't require too much energy. If you're worried about having sex during your pregnancy, talk to your obstetrician to ease your fears. Once your mind is at rest, your body can play.**

As if Deanna's lack of sexual desire weren't enough to contend with, Marcus began contending with his own block: As Deanna's belly grew, so did his "mommy" identity issues. "On the rare occasions that Deanna was willing to have sex, I'd look at her belly and think, Wow, there's a baby in there. It became really difficult to see beyond that and remember she was still my wife."

"Marcus is right that I did tune out," Deanna concedes. "I knew that he was feeling neglected in the bedroom, but

I just put it on the back burner and told myself I'd make it up to him later. Plus, I had resentments of my own. I was the one who was getting fat, throwing up all the time, and worrying myself sick over the baby. And he wanted *me* to take care of *him*? He wanted me to perform obligatory sex when I couldn't go an hour without throwing up? The more I thought about how immature and selfish he was being, the less I wanted to give him any pleasure. I knew that he was seeing me in a different light, too, and that made me feel totally asexual."

The discord grew until the relationship was stretched to its limits. What should have been a happy, bonding time in their marriage became a time of resentment and distance as the couple became physically and emotionally disconnected from each other.

"We were living in one house but in two different worlds," says Marcus. "We were caught up in our own frustrations and weren't thinking about the other person. I know that's true for me. It's bizarre, since we'd finally gotten what we'd always wanted, which was a viable pregnancy. I have many regrets about the way I acted during Deanna's pregnancy. I was selfish a lot of the time, and I know my attitude led to the affair."

It was a Friday morning. Feeling sexually frustrated and forgotten, Marcus left the house. Feeling emotionally neglected, Deanna watched him go. Marcus drove to work, parked his car, and walked into the office. The Other Woman was already there.

"She usually worked downstairs, but she'd recently been transferred to my department," Marcus explains. "I'd known her on a casual basis for a couple years, and she'd always kind of flirted with me, though I hadn't returned her attention. She was a big flirt, and there were rumors she'd slept with more than one guy in the office, but this morning she was particularly flirtatious with me. At least it seemed that way to me, but maybe she wasn't. Maybe I was just seeing what I wanted to see."

According to Marcus, the flirtatious clerk began to dish out some of the attention his wife wasn't serving. When he'd walk into a room, she'd stop what she was doing and make eye contact with him and listen intently to every word that came out of his mouth. She was a fresh face and always smiling, unlike Deanna, who greeted him from the couch, bathrobed, green faced, and growling. And the other woman exuded sexuality, while his wife screamed impending motherhood.

"The other woman always has that advantage," says Marcus. "She gets to put her best face forward, and you don't see all the baggage. It's unfair, unrealistic, and I was too self-absorbed to see through it. She'd smile at me and check me out with her eyes like I was the hottest guy around. By lunchtime, I was thinking things I shouldn't have been, and I was sending vibes back to her."

Having cleared his desk earlier than anticipated, Marcus decided to start the weekend early and leave the office by midafternoon. Little did he know that the new clerk was tracking his path.

"She stopped me in the stairwell on the way down to the parking lot and asked me if I wanted to go for a drink," says Marcus. "You know the sad part? At the moment she stopped me, I was thinking about surprising Deanna by coming home early and taking her for ice cream. I remember standing on the step and thinking about what I was going to do. I know all cheaters say it, but I'd do anything to have that moment back, to take back what I did. All I thought about was instant gratification."

The gratification may have been instant, but it didn't last long. "I found out from another wife," says Deanna, "the wife of Marcus's business associate. The gossip got back to her a week or so later, and one morning she just showed up on my doorstep. She was in tears. She said she'd spent days agonizing over whether to tell me. I knew what she was going to say before she got the words out. Marcus had been acting strange since it happened, and I knew something had changed."

Like many women, Deanna had always sworn that if a man cheated on her, she'd leave. But with her first child only two months away, it wasn't that easy anymore. She knew her decision to stay or go would affect the rest of her life and her daughter's life, so she forced herself to think the situation out.

"I had to do some real soul searching," says Deanna, "and I didn't like everything I found. I realized that our problems were nothing new and that I'd always had a tendency to push Marcus to the sidelines of my life. I realized I had a history of using him for what I needed, then pushing him aside when I didn't need him. That was the case with sex even before I became pregnant, but it was the case in other areas, too. I'm not making excuses for him, but when there are two people in a relationship, both have to look at the roles they play. We talked a lot about the kind of marriage and family we wanted and how we could get there."

"No man has begged for forgiveness like I did," says Marcus. "On my hands and knees. I did everything she said, and for the first time in my life I did it without thinking about myself. The other woman transferred. I talked to our priest; I kept my cell phone in my jacket pocket so she could call me at any time to find out where I was. It took almost losing it all to make me realize how much I had and to make me grow up. I don't know who was more broken-hearted, me or her. I'd totally betrayed her, but looking at my wife's face also broke my heart. There she was, out to there with my baby, and I was screwing around. That's not how my parents raised me. That's not how I want to raise my child."

Eventually, Deanna decided to give Marcus another chance. She knew that he was remorseful and truly believed he would not make the same mistake again. It was a conscious, deliberate decision to stay, but her emotions wouldn't fall in line.

"I wanted to make it work," says Deanna. "On the one hand I wanted to have sex with him because I knew he was missing it, but whenever we'd get close, the tape in my head would start playing. I'd see them together, having sex. I'd hear them groaning. It was graphic, and I was obsessed with the details. What was she wearing? Where did they do it? In what position? Did they do it more than once? Did she suck him? I can't tell you how disgusting it is to have those pictures in your head. My emotions swung to extremes. One minute I'd want to hold and forgive him, and the next I hated him. If I thought about pleasing him sexually, even with a quick hand job, it seemed like I was betraying myself or that I was saying everything was forgiven."

For Deanna and Marcus, the physical and emotional disconnection in their relationship seemed irreparable. Despite their desire to stay together and work things out, they simply couldn't find a way back to intimacy. Yet the path was about to present itself in the most effortless of ways.

"We were sitting on the couch watching television," says Deanna. "I was worrying, as usual, when Marcus slid closer to me and put his hands on my shoulders."

"Her face was tense, and I could tell she was off in another world, worrying about the baby or us. I wanted to make her relax. It seemed like a natural thing to do, so I started to rub her shoulders. I wasn't asking for anything. I just wanted to touch my wife and make her feel better."

Touch can be very healing. Whether the pain is physical, psychological, or emotional, human touch has the potential to lessen suffering. Physical touch can also act as an emotional bridge, a way to cross the distance between two people and bring them closer together. That's what it did for Deanna and Marcus.

> **Studies have shown that the sleep patterns, weight gain, and mental development of infants are improved by early touch. Kangaroo Care is a special form of touch designed for premature babies, where a naked preemie is nestled against the bare skin of its parent. This special form of touch therapy facilitates child-parent bonding and soothes the infant.**

"It felt good having his hands on me again," says Deanna. "We went into the bedroom, and he gave me a full-body massage. It was the first time in months that I felt completely at ease, not just in my own mind but also in his presence. The rest of the world didn't exist. It was just us, touching and talking quietly."

"I could feel Deanna's body relaxing. I could even see her expression softening. The next day I stopped at a holistic store and bought some massage oil they recommended for calming pregnant women, and I started to give her a massage every night. I knew after the first massage that it was going to be our way to reconnect."

Like lovemaking, physical touch can be a powerful way to foster affection between two people. Oxytocin, the so-called bonding hormone that is released by the brain during sex, is also released during physical touch. A prolonged sensual massage session between disconnected lovers is therefore an ideal way to flood the body with feelings of affection, intimacy, and love.

"After several nights of Marcus touching me, I started to feel drawn to him, and drawn to his body again," explains Deanna. "It all progressed very naturally. The closer we got to each other, the further away everybody else, including the other woman, got."

Eventually, the sensual touch turned sexual.

"Deanna was lying on her back, and I was touching her stomach," says Marcus. "She was so sexy, and once in a while I could feel the baby move against my hand. I'd never felt so in love with her. She started caressing my groin, and then stroking. I wasn't expecting it, but she gave me a wonderful hand job. That was the beginning, and it wasn't too long after that that we started to have intercourse again."

"I couldn't have intercourse right away," admits Deanna. "I wasn't ready for that, but I wanted to make him feel as good as he was making me feel. That in itself was a big turning point in our relationship. If both of us had worked at staying connected in the first place, the affair wouldn't have happened. Touch now keeps us close physically and emotionally. We hug a lot more than we used to, and erotic massage is a big part of our love life. Now I feel like nobody can get through the wall we've built around our relationship."

Whether you're on the road to relationship repair or you're just practicing preventative maintenance, set aside a night to experience sensual massage with your man. Choose a night that you don't expect any distractions. To begin, empty the house. Send the kids to Grandma's (okay, at least send them to bed), turn off the phone and the lights, and break out the candles. Turn up the thermostat so your bedroom is toasty. If you have an electric blanket, set it to low-medium and cover it with a sheet or towels for your partner to lie on. Toss towels or sheets into the dryer to warm them up and have a couple of rolled towels ready for head, neck, and knee support.

> If you don't have an electric blanket to lie on, dig out that old heating pad and tuck it under the bedsheets instead. It's an easy way to bring cozy warmth to a massage.

For a more romantic ambience, play some classical music. You want to be connecting with your partner, not singing along with a top-ten pop song. If you wish to incorporate pornography into the sensual massage experience—as we suggested in chapter 18—have a movie or even a website ready for viewing in your bedroom. There are many adult movies that fall under the guise of "sensual massage for couples," and they're a tame way to begin. If you don't want or aren't ready for the visual aspect, cover the television with a towel and just listen to the sexy sounds as background until your curiosity compels you to peek.

The type of product you use to massage your partner depends on the amount of time and money you wish to invest in sensual touch. At the very least, you should have a lightly scented lotion (tangerine and green tea are two of our favorites) to use on your man's body and a personal lubricant to use on his genitals (this is an opportune time to use that warming lube). If the body lotion is unscented, burn incense or a scented candle.

To kick things up a notch and get the most out of this erotic encounter, stock aromatherapy in your arsenal of arousal. Because essential oils come in all scents and flavors, stop by a holistic store and ask for advice if you're a newbie. Staff in these shops are characteristically helpful and extremely knowledgeable, and you'll find the presence of scents can have a more powerful impact on mood than you anticipated. For example, grapefruit is refreshing, while lavender is calming. An essential-oils specialist can also mix different oils to create one that perfectly suits your needs and tastes. Our longtime personal favorite is ambrosia. Delicious.

An easy option is to purchase a complete massage kit, again from a love shop or online. If you have the chance, it's best to shop in person so you can benefit from an honest face-to-face recommendation from the salesperson. A basic massage kit will include a selection of essential oils and sometimes a lubricant, but others also include sensual massage videos, feathers, and massagers and vibrators. Some even boast attachments to caress your partner inside and out.

Now that your bedroom is a passion parlor, your bed is a sexy spa table, and all your accessories are ready for action, ask your man to have a quick shower—solo or partnered—and to brush his teeth before he joins you in the bedroom. If he has all his personal grooming done before you start, he can drift off to sleep after the massage is over. When he's squeaky clean, have him lie naked, facedown, on the warmed blanket or towels. Tuck a pillow or a thick, rolled towel underneath his upper body to raise his shoulders off the bed. This will let him rest his head on his forehead and keep his head straight, rather than cranked to the side. It'll also make it easier for you to work on his shoulders. You can also tuck rolled towels under the front of his ankles to similarly support his feet and help him relax his legs.

Remember that you're going to perform sensual massage, not therapeutic massage, so don't become preoccupied with textbook technique, sequencing, or the strength of your strokes. If your man has a sore back or muscle injury, he needs a certified massage therapist. Otherwise, he needs his woman, and you don't need a certificate to touch him in an erotically relaxing way. Use your instincts to get a sense of what he likes. Concentrate on slow, purposeful, sensual strokes and use artistic license with the directions suggested in this chapter. Different men will prefer different things, so be sure to communicate during the session. After all, this lube job is about connecting. Finally, be aware of your own limits and use your body weight to lean into your man's body as you stroke rather than rely on your upper-body strength.

Ready to rub? First, find a position that you're comfortable in. This depends on your preference and on your relative body size. You can kneel by his side, straddle his body panty free so he can feel your nakedness, or kneel by his head. In any case, you'll likely be changing positions as the massage progresses. Start by synchronizing your respiration until you and your man are breathing in time. This may not last long, but it'll slip you into the same groove and force you to consciously relax. Next, place your fingertips on your partner's scalp and lightly rake them down his head, neck, and back, continuing down over his buttocks and legs to his feet. Start at the top again and rake your fingertips down his arms. This first contact simply awakens his body as a whole, so repeat it as many times as you wish.

Stiffen your fingers and rub your partner's scalp harder to get his circulation going. Pretend that you're giving him a power shampoo. Gently scratch his scalp with your fingernails. Now take some of your massage oil and rub it between your hands to generate warmth. You're not going to stroke with any pressure yet, you're just going to apply the oil to his body. Smooth the oil over the top of his shoulders, all the way down his back, buttocks, and legs, then back up to his shoulders again. Spread the oil down his arms.

With a slow and deliberate motion, begin to knead the top of your man's shoulders with as much pressure as he likes or as you're comfortable using. Tell him to close his eyes, exhale, and consciously focus on relaxing his muscles. (I sometimes tell Don to visualize a tight ball of string slowly loosening and then unraveling.) Fan your flattened hands outward and rub his shoulder blades and upper back with smaller circular strokes. Use palm strokes and thumb strokes to relax his shoulders and shoulder blades.

Lean into his body and slide your flattened hands downward on either side of his spine to his lower back. Be careful not to apply pressure directly on his spine. When you reach his buttocks, fan your hands outward to his sides and pull your hands back up along the sides of his body. Repeat this pattern—down his back and up along his sides—as many times as you wish.

Starting at the top of his spine, make a peace sign with your fingers and place the pads of your index and middle fingers on either side of his spine. Rake your stiff fingers down his back in this V shape, with a finger pad on each side of his spine and again being careful to not apply direct pressure on his backbone. Go all the way down to his buttocks. Make smaller circling strokes on his buttocks with your flattened hands, then use your fingers to knead them. Be aware of how smoothly your hands are moving over his skin and use more oil if there's any friction.

Because limbs are usually massaged upward, toward the heart, don't continue down his thighs. Instead, begin at his ankles and move upward to his thighs, stroking and kneading the back of his legs until you reach his buttocks. Slide both your hands up over his buttocks and keep stroking upward over his back, on either side of his spine, finally reaching his upper back and shoulders. Rather than continuing down his arms, start at his wrists and move upward to his shoulders with stroking and kneading motions.

Treat your man to a few more broad strokes down his back and up along his sides, perhaps again raking the muscles on either side of his spine with stiff fingers. Because we hold so much of our stress and tension in our neck and shoulders, you may want to return to the top of his shoulders and knead them for a while longer as well. Keep reminding your man to breathe regularly and to visualize his muscle fibers relaxing. (That ball of string should be coming apart by now.) And, as always, be conscious of how easily your hands glide over him. A good lube job is friction free, so don't be thrifty with the oil.

Finish this facedown massage by applying long, feathery fingertip strokes from head to toe. He should barely be able to feel these.

> If your partner likes a more invigorating massage, add a chopping motion (using the sides of your hands) or a pummeling motion (using loose fists) to loosen up his back muscles. Again, never work directly over his spine.

When you're ready for the flip side, ask your partner to roll over and lie on his back. Place one rolled towel under his neck and another under both his knees for support. Starting at the top of his shoulders, smooth warmed massage oil down his arms to his hands, then down his chest and abdomen. Spread the oil over his hips and down his legs to his feet. Don't touch his groin area yet, even if he hints you missed a spot. Sensual touch will slip into sexual soon enough.

Begin by massaging his face. Move up along his jaw line with your fingers to his temples and massage them in a circular motion. Use your thumb pads to lightly stroke outward over his cheekbones to his temples, then put your thumbs together between his eyes and sweep your thumbs up and over his forehead. Pinch his eyebrows softly along their length. Don's favorite move is the one in which I hold his ears and very gently pull on them. First, I pull outward on the lobe, and then I hold the top of his ear between my thumb and fingers and move the entire ear in small circles. You can also finger-stroke the groove behind the ear. Follow the face massage by rubbing and scratching his scalp.

Drag your fingertips down the sides of your partner's neck and knead the tops of his shoulders. Slide your hands down and gently stroke his chest outward to his sides, moving down his rib cage as you go. Now place your hands on one side of his body and pull upward. This is easiest if you're kneeling on the bed opposite the side you're working on, leaning over his body. As you pull up on his side, sit back down on your heels. Finally, place your hands on his chest again and stroke outward to his shoulders with gentle pressure, using as much oil as is necessary.

Now take each of your partner's hands and arms in turn and massage in an upward direction. Hold his hand in yours and use your thumbs to stroke from his wrist to his fingertips. The palm of the hand is particularly responsive to massage, so spend some time stroking and kneading this spot. Slide your fingers between his so you're in an interlocking handhold—this might be a sweet time to give him a deep kiss on the mouth—and then continue up his arm. Use a combination of long strokes and a wringing motion to massage his arms up to his shoulders.

Drag your hands down his chest to his abdomen, and massage his belly with large circles in a clockwise direction, using plenty of oil. Run your hands down along his hips. You're forgiven if you accidentally brush against something you shouldn't.

To massage the front of his legs, start at the ankles and use long, well-oiled upward strokes to his thighs. Again, if your fingertips were to inadvertently touch his testicles or perineum, he probably wouldn't request another masseuse. So practice a little malpractice.

Now apply sexy squeezes to each of his feet in turn. Use your thumbs to stroke his soles, moving from heel to toes. Pull each of his toes and then slip your fingers through his toes so that your fingers and his toes are interlocking. Slide your fingers out, then slip them through again before returning to stroke his soles with your thumbs. Cradle his foot in your hand and tell him to relax his ankle as you gently circle the joint through its range of motion. Return to rub the sole again before setting his foot down on the bed.

Finish this face-up massage the same way that you finished the facedown: by applying long, feathery strokes along the length of his body and limbs, using just your fingertips.

Okay, it's the moment we've all been waiting for: the genital massage. The lubrication you use on your partner's genitals will depend on what you've stocked. Some products are fine for genital use, so you can continue on your current course; however, if you're at all uncertain, clean your hands and use a standard personal lubricant. Warm the lube between your hands and apply it first to your partner's testicles, massaging his scrotum and gently pulling it away from his body.

Caress your man's perineum, then slide your hand under and over his scrotum, continuing in a single stroke up along the underside of his shaft. Place your hand or fingers around the base of his penis and lightly stroke upward on his shaft. When he's hard, you can adopt a down-and-up stroke, maybe adding a twist to your wrist when you get to the head of his penis. (Incidentally, I've found this to be an ideal point in the massage to casually mention any large purchases you may have recently made.) Don't forget his testicles as you stroke his shaft—bounce them in one hand while the other strokes. Putting pressure on his perineum during stroking also increases pleasure, so push a thumb against this sensitive spot while your pumping hand moves up and down his penis.

Delayed gratification is the guiding principle of genital massage. The more times you can bring your partner close to orgasm but stop before he actually climaxes, the stronger his sexual release will ultimately be. Accordingly, the pressure, rhythm, variety, and pace of your strokes depend on how well you can read your man and how long you want to make this lube job last. It also depends on how you want this massage session to end. Do you want to bring him to orgasm with a hand job, or do you want to give him the full-body treatment and proceed to intercourse? If you choose to finish with a hand job, instruct your man to maintain a deep and regular breathing pattern during his orgasm to increase its intensity and immerse himself in the wave of pleasure.

If you decide to complete his experience with sexual intercourse, straddle his body (facing his head or his feet) in the woman-on-top position, and lower yourself onto him. Tell him to relax, breathe through it, and lose himself in the feelings as you do all the work. It's all part of the sensual massage package, and you're a very comprehensive masseuse.

After your session is over, spend some time lying quietly next to your partner. If he wants to drift off to sleep, let him. There are few states of mind and body as perfectly blissful as that following a sensual massage, so let your man soak in the serenity.

Adding sensual massage to your love life has great potential to strengthen the intimate connection between you and your man. It also offers opportunities for ongoing variety. There are countless massage oils and lubricants you can use in your sessions to keep them as fresh as they are familiar. Another way to add something new to the experience is to incorporate hot-stone therapy into sensual massage. While this ancient healing therapy has recently enjoyed a revival in spas across the world, it's an easy and exquisite way to bring a new dimension to your intimate massage sessions at home, too.

Hot-stone therapy is the process of placing heated stones on specific places on the body, either directly on the skin or on a cloth. For example, stones of varying sizes may be placed on the back, on the limbs, on the face, in the palms of the hands, and between the toes. As the heat from the stone penetrates the body, muscle knots and tension are dissolved. But stone therapy has more than a physical effect, as the heat and presence of the stones can lull a person into a deep state of emotional tranquillity and peace. The practice therefore creates an ideal state of body and mind in which to connect physically and emotionally with your man.

Like sensual-massage kits, complete hot-stone-therapy massage kits are also available. Some come with just the basics (a number of smooth basalt stones); others may include a warmer and tongs for the stones, essential oils, and either an instructional book or video that will show you exactly where the stones are to be placed on the body. Or, you may wish to visit a rock and gem specialty store and choose your own stones individually. Considering the popularity of hot-stone therapy, the staff are likely well versed in the practice and will be able to advise you which stones to select.

Although you should be able to buy a decent starter set of stones (whether in a kit or individually) for the price of a night out for two, don't be too frugal with your purchase. Stones of lesser quality, such as those included in inexpensive kits, cannot hold heat nearly as well as better-quality stones. Take our word for it, these gems are worth the investment. If diamonds are a girl's best friend, hot stones are her lover's.

As we've seen in this chapter, sensual touch is a powerful tool. Not only can it bridge the emotional, physical, and sexual distance between two lovers, it can also help heal a broken relationship. But perhaps most important, sensual massage can help a couple maintain the strength of their loving connection to prevent a breakdown from happening in the first place.

We certainly don't mean to oversimplify intimate emotional and physical issues, whether the problem is infidelity, arguments over pornography, or something else altogether, but the fact remains, it is far better to prevent this type of relationship damage than it is to repair it. And sensual massage may be one way to bring and keep you close as a couple. Remember, an ounce of prevention is worth a pound of cure. Take the time to clear the snow from the wipers before you turn them on. Take the time to stay connected to your partner before your precious bond is compromised.

Part Five

Maintenance Coupons

Lube Job #20

○

Hassle-Free Maintenance Sex Coupons

Throughout this handbook, we've tried to redeem maintenance sex in principle. Now it's your man's turn to redeem it in a more practical sense. Maintenance coupons, which can be exchanged for sexual favors at his pleasure, are a straightforward yet sexy way for your partner to indicate his needs are in need. Cut out these reusable, strictly maintenance sex coupons and give them to your man. Or create and customize your own coupon book by including the quickies or all-nighters he likes best.

If it so happens that your man wants to cash in a coupon (or a combination of coupons!) you'd rather not honor at that particular moment, don't panic. Instead, offer him a friendly rain check and negotiate an alternative exchange: maybe a slow blow job as he watches his favorite television show for that labor-intensive precoital massage or a quickie hand job in the car for that doggy-style romp on the kitchen floor. The compromise is as important as the currency. As long as your man has the means to communicate his needs and an assurance that his needs will be met one way or another, he'll be smiling all the way to the bank.

Maintenance sex coupons are the ultimate gift certificates for men and a user-friendly way to ensure that your partner stays in excellent condition at all times. They're maintenance made easy. Best of all, they show your man that you recognize his sexual needs are legitimate, that you want to lovingly satisfy them, and that you sincerely care about maintaining your emotional and physical connection as a couple.

Maintenance Sex Coupon

**Redeemable for sexual intercourse, initiated by you,
within the next _____ hours**

Maintenance Sex Coupon

Redeemable for one long-lasting genital massage

Maintenance Sex Coupon

**Redeemable for one hand job in the car while
listening to the music of my choice**

Maintenance Sex Coupon

Redeemable for one 69 session on the couch

Maintenance Sex Coupon

**Redeemable for one long French kiss
on any body part of mine**

Maintenance Sex Coupon

**Redeemable for one cock-a-doodle-do
hand job to begin before I wake up**

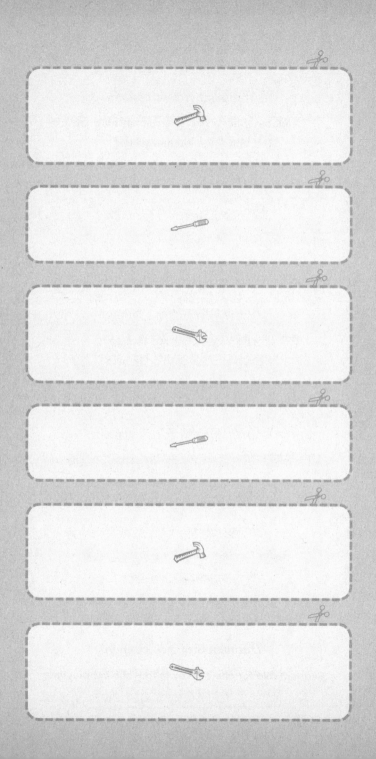

Maintenance Sex Coupon

**Redeemable for one after-dinner blow job
under the kitchen table**

Maintenance Sex Coupon

Redeemable for one blow job performed outdoors

Maintenance Sex Coupon

**Redeemable for one mutual
masturbation session in bed**

Maintenance Sex Coupon

Redeemable for one hand job performed outdoors

Maintenance Sex Coupon

**Redeemable for sexual intercourse
performed outdoors**

Maintenance Sex Coupon

Redeemable for one sex-toy (of my choice) playtime

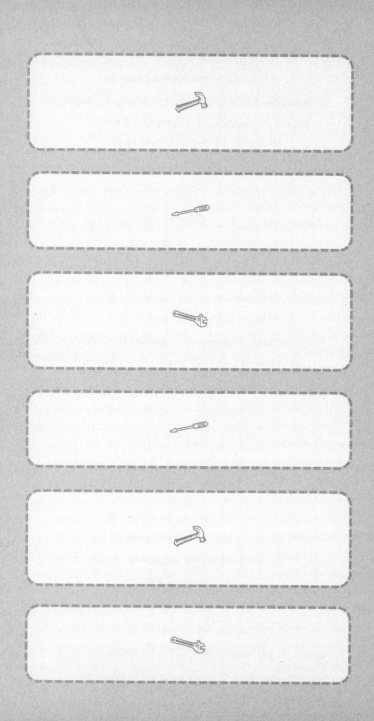

Maintenance Sex Coupon

**Redeemable for one "Mannequin Woman" session,
where you stand or lie completely still and
let me do whatever I want to you**

Maintenance Sex Coupon

Redeemable for one XXX-rated movie night

Maintenance Sex Coupons

**Redeemable for super slick sexual intercourse,
with both our bodies covered in baby oil**

Maintenance Sex Coupon

Redeemable for one X-rated story time session

Maintenance Sex Coupon

**Redeemable for the chance to watch
you masturbate**

Maintenance Sex Coupon

Redeemable for one bedroom striptease

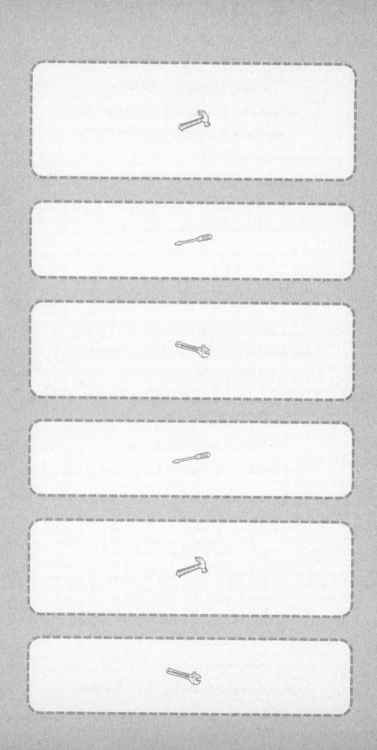

Maintenance Sex Coupon

**Redeemable for one blow job performed
while you sit on the side of the tub**

Maintenance Sex Coupon

Redeemable for one "power polish"

Maintenance Sex Coupon

**Redeemable for sexual intercourse in the
laundry room, with you on top of the washing
machine (on the spin cycle)**

Maintenance Sex Coupon

**Redeemable for sexual intercourse
in front of a mirror**

Maintenance Sex Coupon

**Redeemable for one blindfold
and/or restraints sex session**

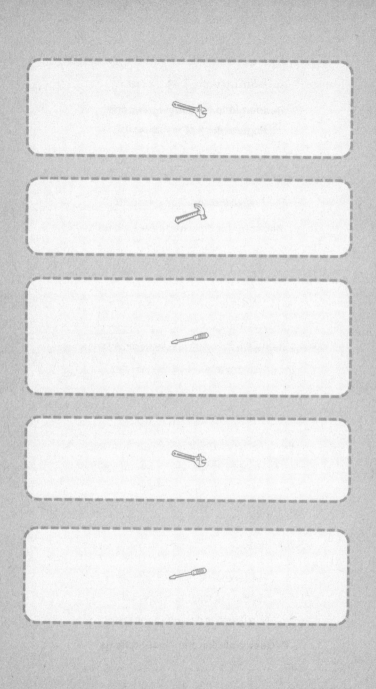

Maintenance Sex Coupon

Redeemable for you to wear one
lingerie item of my choice

Maintenance Sex Coupon

Redeemable for hands-free sexual intercourse,
where we have sex without using our hands to help

Maintenance Sex Coupon

Redeemable for one prolonged necking session

Maintenance Sex Coupon

Redeemable for a long look at your naked body

Maintenance Sex Coupon

Redeemable for one hand job in the shower

Maintenance Sex Coupon

Redeemable for one closet quickie

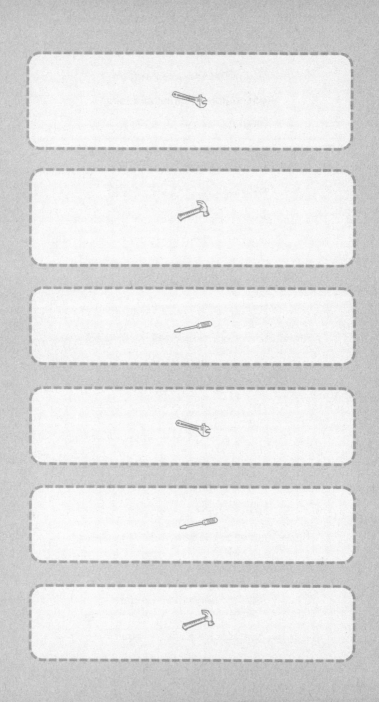

Maintenance Sex Coupon

Redeemable for one lap dance

Maintenance Sex Coupon

**Redeemable for an opportunity
to try something new in bed**

Maintenance Sex Coupon

Maintenance Sex Coupon

Maintenance Sex Coupon

Maintenance Sex Coupon

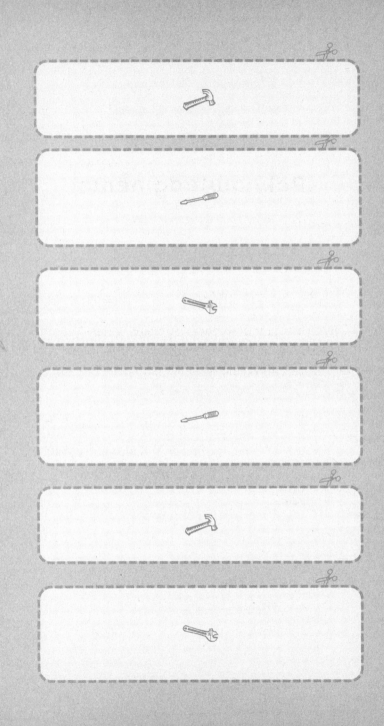

Acknowledgments

Many thanks go out to Susan Raihofer, literary agent extraordinaire with the David Black Agency in New York. Your advice, efforts, and sense of humor have been invaluable to us.

Thanks also to Sara Carder and Kathryn Kimball at Tarcher/Penguin USA for their support and exceptional editorial direction.

Index

About the Authors

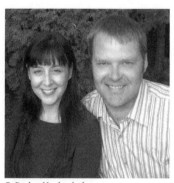

© *Darlene Vandenakerboom*

Maintenance sex saved **Don and Debra Macleod**'s marriage, and *Lube Jobs* is inspired by their journey back to amorous intimacy after the sexual stalemate that followed the premature birth of their son. They are also the authors of *The French Maid*, which has been featured in *USA Today*, in the Style section of *The New York Times*, and on the "Borders Recommends" list. The Macleods live in Alberta, Canada.